EXPLODING THE MYTHS ABOUT ESTROGEN AND MENOPAUSE

MYTH: All menopausal women should have hormone replacement therapy.

FACT: There are medical reasons why some women should *not* be on estrogen.

MYTH: If you don't have hot flashes, insomnia, or other menopausal symptoms, you don't need estrogen.

FACT: There are many health benefits to hormone replacement therapy, in addition to the relief of menopausal symptoms.

MYTH: The risks of going on estrogen are worse than the benefits.

FACT: Statistics show increases in life expectancy for those on estrogen.

ESTROGEN

Answers to All Your Questions
About Hormone
Replacement Therapy and
Natural Alternatives

MARK STOLAR, M.D.

AVON BOOKS ◆ NEW YORK

The ideas, procedures, and suggestions in this book are intended to supplement, not replace, the medical advice of a trained medical professional. All matters regarding your health require medical supervision. Consult your physician before adopting the suggestions in this book, as well as any condition that may require diagnosis or medical attention. The author and publisher disclaim any liability arising directly or indirectly from the use of this book.

AVON BOOKS
A division of
The Hearst Corporation
1350 Avenue of the Americas
New York, New York 10019

Copyright © 1997 by Current Medical Directions, Inc.
Published by arrangement with Current Medical Directions, Inc.
Visit our website at **http://AvonBooks.com**
Library of Congress Catalog Card Number: 97-93168
ISBN: 0-380-79076-9

First Avon Books Printing: September 1997

AVON TRADEMARK REG. U.S. PAT. OFF. AND IN OTHER COUNTRIES, MARCA REGISTRADA, HECHO EN U.S.A.

Printed in the U.S.A.

WCD   10   9   8   7   6   5   4   3   2

Contents

ESTROGEN

ONE

Hormones and Their Role in Your Body

CASE STUDY

Allison, a 57-year-old postal employee, seemed a little embarrassed during our initial visit, and it took several minutes of friendly conversation before she felt comfortable enough to talk about what was troubling her—a sudden loss of libido.

"I still love my husband very much," she explained, "but my sex drive has all but disappeared. I enjoy cuddling, but I have almost no desire for intercourse." She was experiencing vaginal dryness, and most attempts at sex were painful. "Is this something I'm just going to have to live with?" she asked.

Like many women her age, Allison was under the impression that a loss of libido was a natural part of the aging process. This is a common myth. A sudden decrease in sex drive usually indicates a physical or psychological condition, and in Allison's case I was fairly certain it was hormonal in origin.

Based on her medical history, I suspected that most of Allison's complaints, specifically loss of libido and painful intercourse, were caused by the onset of menopause and the resulting depletion of estrogen—a fact confirmed through a blood test. During a follow-up visit, I explained to Allison exactly what was happening to her body, and prescribed estrogen. I also suggested she use a vaginal lubricant to make sex a little more comfortable until her body adjusted to the hormone replacement.

Three weeks later, Allison reported that she was feeling much better, and that her desire for sex had returned.

In order to better understand what estrogen and other hormones are and how they function, it helps to know a little about the "bigger picture" known as your endocrine system. The endocrine system is your body's biological communications and control center. It is a network of organs and glands that secretes hormones (think of hormones as chemical message carriers) to other areas of the body in order to regulate a variety of body functions. In women, this network includes the ovaries, the thyroid gland, the pituitary gland, the adrenal glands, the pancreas, the thymus, and the hypothalamus. The various hormones affect aspects of reproduction and growth (for example, puberty, pregnancy, and menopause), digestion, bone building and strength, the burning of calories, the regulation of body temperature, metabolism, and maintenance of the body's fluid and salt balance.

The endocrine system works something like this. Once a hormone is produced by an organ or gland, it is sent through the bloodstream to a specific receptor on another organ or gland. These chemical messages either turn on or turn off—or speed up or slow down—the organ's functions. For example, when a young woman reaches puberty, the hypothalamus—the part of the brain that controls functions such as sleep, body temperature, and reproductive processes—signals the pituitary gland to release a hormone that ultimately stimulates the production of estrogen in the ovaries. This in turn results in breast development and the growth of pubic hair, among other changes. The endocrine system is complex. Sometimes a problem in one part of it can cause trouble in another part—for example, hot flashes are triggered by a drop in estrogen which upsets the hypothalamus's ability to regulate temperature properly. Other times, one endocrine gland may compensate partially for another. After menopause, for example, when the ovaries stop making estrogen, the adrenal glands may produce some in lesser amounts. When your body is functioning properly, just the right levels and kinds of hormones are produced at just the right time.

Today, women have available to them an enormous amount of information about the endocrine system and hormones like estrogen, some of which was unknown to medical science until only several years ago. Not until the 1980s was there even a medical specialty that focused solely on women's endocrine systems and reproductive health, and researchers are discovering new information about the endocrine system every day. When your mother reached menopause, doctors probably knew less than 1 percent of what they now know about women's hormones and reproductive biology. The birth control pill became available only in the early 1960s, and using hormone therapy to replace depleted estrogen has only recently been considered standard therapy.

There is still much that doctors do not know about estrogen and its role in your body, but many questions can be answered with confidence. This is important if you want to take advantage of this knowledge in order to make informed decisions about your health.

Q: What is estrogen?
A: Estrogen is referred to as a "female" sex hormone. It is closely associated with a woman's reproductive life, and larger amounts of it occur in women than in men. There are actually three estrogens: estradiol, estriol, and estrone. Although the three estrogens differ a little in their chemical structure, that is not as important as where they are made and when they are most active. Estradiol is the "main" estrogen, produced in the ovaries. Estradiol is active from puberty to menopause. Estriol is made in the placenta, and is most active during pregnancy. Estrone is made in fat tissue and is the chief source of estrogen after menopause. All three estrogens derive from

progesterone, another female sex hormone that, in women, prepares the uterus for the reception and development of the fertilized egg. Doctors measure estradiol to determine estrogen levels, since it is most often involved in estrogen deficiency conditions. In men, the testes also produce estrogen, although in significantly lower amounts.

Q: I've heard that estrogen affects almost every single part of my body. How?

A: A normal level of estrogen is needed for general good health. But more specifically, estrogen has these rather wide and varied effects: It keeps your skin supple and your hair full and healthy, influences certain brain chemicals, stimulates breast development and the rounding of thighs and buttocks in puberty, helps maintain the density of your spine and other bones, prepares your uterus for pregnancy, and lubricates the vagina.

Q: How is estrogen involved in regulating body temperature?

A: The entire endocrine system is involved, with estrogen playing a crucial role as the means of communication. The skin and the nervous system together sense changes in body temperature, and estrogen carries the message to the hypothalamus, which in turn directs us to shiver to generate heat or sweat to cool off. When estrogen levels drop at menopause, the balance between the hypothalamus and the nervous system is upset, so temperature regulation is not always properly maintained.

Q: Does estrogen keep the skin young?
A: Up to a point, yes. Age and exposure to too much ultraviolet light will do their damage regardless. But natural estrogen circulating internally in your body does make your skin look and feel healthy. If your estrogen level is too low, your skin may look dull. The reason is that estrogen regulates the lubricating oil produced by the sebaceous glands, which are located along hair shafts all over the body. If these glands become overactive for one reason or another, you may develop acne. If high levels of androgen are the cause—androgen is a "male" sex hormone—some specialists recommend using estrogen in the form of contraceptive pills to combat these troubling skin conditions.

Q: How does estrogen affect risk of heart disease?
A: It appears to prevent buildup of plaque in blood vessel walls. Plaque makes these walls narrow and increases the risk of heart attack. Women have thus always had an advantage over men as far as having healthy hearts. But many doctors have been concerned that women's changing lifestyles may narrow that gap; in particular, many more women have taken up cigarette smoking in the past few decades. The good news is that smoking is now on the decline.

Q: Does estrogen have anything to do with my mood swings?

A: It definitely could, although you should also consider whether your diet, stress level, or overwork may be contributing. It also depends on whether your mood swings are due to premenstrual syndrome or to the onset of menopause. Estrogen has powerful effects on the brain (as do progesterone, androgens, and thyroid hormones). There are specific receptors in the brain (just as there are in the breast and other areas affected by this hormone) to which estrogen attaches, triggering various changes. For example, estrogen can modify the structure of certain nerve cells so that they make more and better connections with other cells. It can make cells in the brain become more responsive to chemicals that carry messages to the brain—for example, those that stimulate feelings of pleasure. So changes in estrogen's activity could influence your mood strongly. But if you are going through menopause, you may also not be getting enough sleep because of hot flashes—brief episodes of rapid heartbeat and sweating—or you may be worried about how menopause will affect your life.

Q: Is premenstrual syndrome due to low estrogen?

A: Premenstrual syndrome is not exactly due to low estrogen. Low estrogen does impair the brain's ability to regulate mood. But some women suffer premenstrual syndrome even though they have perfectly healthy levels of estrogen. The answer lies in the complicated relationship between the brain, estrogen, and progesterone, which also affects brain chemistry. Some women may just have a difference in the makeup of their brain receptors, so that they react more or less strongly to changes in levels of estrogen and progesterone.

Q: Is estrogen an appetite suppressant?
A: That is a common theory that surfaces from time to time and then loses popularity again. The idea is that the weight gain often associated with premenstrual syndrome—and with the menopause—is due to decline in estrogen levels. There is no scientific evidence linking estrogen to changes in weight during the menstrual cycle. As for menopause, it is true that many women gain a few pounds at that time. What is interesting is not the weight so much as the change in fat distribution. Estrogen rounds out the body at puberty; after menopause, fat often declines in the "round parts"—the hips, buttocks, and breasts—and moves to the upper body and shoulders or to the abdomen. This might be accompanied by some weight gain or simply by a feeling of being heavier because you are carrying weight in different places.

Q: Does estrogen affect intelligence?
A: It has been reported that in the second week after menstruation, when estrogen levels are at their peak, women do best on tests of verbal acuity, perceptual speed, and fine motor coordina-

tion. And we know that estrogen does stimulate nerve functioning and communication in the brain. It has even been suggested that declining estrogen is the reason for the short-term memory loss sometimes experienced at menopause. But there is no solid information to support these beliefs. It is possible that women test better the second week after menstruation because they simply feel better at that time of the month than they do just before or during menstruation, thus their energies are free for mental activity—or what doctors call "cognitive function." People have studied cognitive function in postmenopausal women to see if hormone replacement therapy (HRT), which is usually a combination of estrogen and progestin, made a difference. So far, it looks as if keeping good functioning, or suffering a decline with age, has very little to do with estrogen and much more to do with genetics and other factors.

Q: **My doctor can't explain medically why I'm not feeling very well, don't have my usual energy, don't sleep well, and have aches in my joints. Could estrogen deficiency explain it? I'm at the menopausal age but I'm still having my periods and haven't had any hot flashes.**

A: Yes. Women react differently to the decline in ovarian activity and the loss of estrogen that begin a long time—sometimes several years—before the initial symptoms of menopause appear. Sometimes you can only be sure that lack of estrogen is the problem if you try some hormone replacement and the symptoms go away.

Q: How much estrogen should I have?
A: Tests for estrogen levels measure the number of picograms of estradiol (an extremely small quantity) per milliliter of your blood (about a fifth of a teaspoon). During your reproductive years (but not while you are pregnant) you probably have 40 to 600 pg/ml, the lowest levels occurring just before and after menstruation. During pregnancy the level soars to 15,000 to 30,000 pg/ml. Some experts put 70 pg/ml (the amount a man has in his bloodstream) as the minimum amount needed by women; others put it at 60. Somewhere between 60 and 70 is the level at which you may suffer menopausal symptoms or lose protection against osteoporosis—a disease in which bones become brittle. You need about 100 pg/ml to keep your heart healthy. Thus, a level of 60 to 150 is generally acceptable.

Q: How do I find out if I have enough estrogen?
A: Laboratory tests are done on a very small sample of blood drawn from inside your elbow. Your doctor may ask to draw blood again after he has seen the results of the first test, because the results may contradict his reading of your symptoms and he may suspect a laboratory error. It is a difficult test to perform, and not all labs are equally efficient. Also, the results may suggest to him that the test is inaccurate because of the time of day your blood was drawn. Hormone levels

go up and down a lot over a twenty-four-hour period; for example, levels of testosterone, a male sex hormone, go way down in the afternoon. Estradiol levels fluctuate more than any other hormone.

Q: How do estrogen receptors work?
A: Sex hormones do not do anything active until they connect with certain proteins located on their "target" organs—that is, the organs they regulate or influence. For example, when the ovaries start making estrogen at puberty, it travels to the breast, where it attaches to estrogen receptors. This "turns on" the breast's built-in capacity for growth. Long before puberty, we have all the essential ingredients—the tissues, glands, and hormones—for every part of our reproductive life. They are just not activated until the appropriate time.

Q: Why do my breasts get full and feel tender at the beginning of my period?
A: The ovaries are producing a lot more estrogen than usual. This increases blood flow to the breasts, so they do not just feel fuller, they really are fuller. Since the breasts do not stretch to hold the extra fluid, they become tight and tender. The extra blood supply also may make them feel much warmer than usual.

Q: What determines when menstruation begins?
A: Various hormones—including pituitary gland hormones and androgen—are involved. But no-

body really knows why menstruation begins exactly when it does. Some experts argue that it may be prompted by reaching the body weight necessary to carry a pregnancy, and they suggest that this may explain why young women with anorexia often begin menstruation later than usual. But there are some things that contradict this theory—for example, some girls who are naturally very small and thin have normal periods at a normal age. What we do know is that at some point, the hypothalamus signals the pituitary gland to release a hormone called gonadotropin, which instructs the ovaries to start producing estrogen. This stimulates the development of the uterus, breasts, pubic hair, and all the other changes of puberty.

Q: I've heard of polycystic breasts, but what are polycystic ovaries?
A: The ovaries contain pocketlike follicles that release eggs for fertilization. Polycystic ovaries occur when follicles growing just under the ovary surface do not erupt to make the eggs available for fertilization. The follicles stay under the surface and keep being produced as the pituitary gland does not get the proper signal: "Follicles have erupted, stop producing any more." The ovaries fill with tiny cysts (unerupted follicles). This causes irregular periods, infertility, abnormal hair growth, and weight gain, which can be treated with hormones that stimulate development of a normal cycle.

Q: **I thought all hormones were sex hormones and had to do with reproduction. What do the others do?**

A: All hormones—including the sex hormones—carry chemical messages from the organs that manufacture them to the organs they influence. They turn on or off—or speed up or slow down—these organs' activities. For example, they help extract nutrients from the foods we eat and control the burning or storing of calories. They regulate the body's fluid balance, the formation of bones, and the growth and activity of muscles. There are still some things we do not know about how hormones work, and new ones are still being discovered from time to time. We do know that we cannot live or be healthy without them—and, for the most part, they do their jobs well.

Q: **Do men and women really have the same kinds of sex hormones?**

A: Essentially. There are several male sex hormones or androgens, the ones of most importance to women being testosterone and androstenedione. The female sex hormones, in addition to progesterone, are the three estrogens—estradiol, estriol, and estrone. In fact, all sex hormones are derived from progesterone. The testes make female hormones as well as male. The ovaries make testosterone as well as estrogen, and women's adrenal glands also make testosterone. The difference between the sexes is in how much of each hormone they have. For example, a woman's testosterone level is usually about a tenth as much as a man's.

Q: Is it true that a male hormone gives women their sex drive? If so, does it decline after menopause like estrogen?

A: Testosterone is the only hormone to influence women's libido or sex drive. What is interesting is that, with the onset of menopause, the ovaries produce less and less estrogen, but they keep on producing testosterone. The level of circulating or "free" testosterone, the most active kind, may even be a little higher than it was premenopausally. So there is no biological reason for reduced sex drive after menopause—and many women find that their libido increases. But hormones are only part of the story. Women's sexual desire involves a whole complex of physical, psychological, and social factors. There could be many nonhormonal reasons why a woman's interest in sex changes in either direction after menopause. Painful intercourse due to thinning and drying of the vaginal membranes, for example, is a common problem.

Q: What do sex hormones have to do with bones becoming brittle?

A: Bones may seem solid and inert, but actually they are constantly in a state of change. Bone builds up, gets broken down, and new bone is built. It takes a well-balanced endocrine system to orchestrate these activities, and a number of hormones contribute to it. But estrogen plays a key role. It smooths the way for vitamin D and calcium to do their work in bone buildup. It also keeps the bone-dissolving process in check so it does not outrun bone-making.

Q: Since I was in my fifties, I have not had to shave my legs or underarms. Does that mean I have a hormone deficiency of some kind?

A: Levels of male hormones, which usually stimulate hair growth in those areas, naturally decline in the premenopausal and menopausal years. This is not considered a "deficiency" unless there are other more striking problems or symptoms. Just enjoy the convenience.

Q: Men don't seem to stop making their hormones; why don't women keep on making estrogen for life?

A: To be precise, estrogen is manufactured in the egg cells of the ovary. When you are born, you already have all the eggs you are ever going to have—about 400,000 of them. After puberty, every month between twenty and one thousand eggs mature and are ready for fertilization; usually only one is actually released by the ovary at ovulation. All the rest die off, and so does that one if it is not fertilized. This means that eventually, after enough menstrual periods, the ovary has essentially run out of eggs, which are the stimulus for estrogen production. The generally accepted idea is that we are programmed so that we cannot produce any more babies after we have reached an age when they might not be as healthy as those produced when we are young.

Q: What are FSH and LH? Are they hormones, too?

A: Yes, but they are called pituitary hormones because they are made in that gland, not in the reproductive system. FSH stands for follicle stimulating hormone; LH is luteinizing hormone. They are intimately involved with a woman's reproductive life. Menstrual cycles have three major phases. The first, at the beginning two weeks of the cycle, is called the "follicular" phase. The hypothalamus signals the pituitary gland that it is time to release FSH. This stimulates the ovarian follicles—which contain your eggs—to begin developing. FSH also encourages the follicles to release more estrogen than usual. This sends a message right back to the hypothalamus to rush out some LH, and that causes the eggs to be released. This second stage of the menstrual cycle is called the luteal phase. Then the follicle changes into a structure called the corpus luteum, or "yellow body," whose job at that point is to make progesterone. Progesterone does a variety of things to prepare the uterus for pregnancy. If fertilization of eggs does not occur, the decline in LH and estrogen leads to the next stage, which is menstruation itself. The uterus sheds its special "egg ready" lining to be cleared for the next possible pregnancy.

Q: **What makes the endocrine system so much more important for women than for men?**

A: Women have much more complicated reproductive lives, which are regulated by hormones from before puberty to after menopause. Hormones direct the onset of menstruation and the sexual changes that go with it. They stimulate the follicles deep within the ovaries to grow, ripen, and release eggs, to ready the uterus for pregnancy, and to prepare for the next monthly cycle if there is no fertilization. It is an endocrine gland—the pituitary—that signals milk production to start after childbirth. Finally, the endocrine system decides when it is time to phase out reproduction; then it also influences what symptoms—if any—a woman has during her change of life. The endocrine system is also one factor in susceptibility or resistance to breast cancer, heart disease, and osteoporosis.

Q: **I've heard the ovary called "the unique endocrine." What does that mean?**

A: It is the only endocrine gland that does not function for life.

TWO

~∞~

Estrogen and Menopause

CASE STUDY

"At first, I assumed my melancholy was just one of the many mood swings I was experiencing as a result of menopause," said Betty, a 54-year-old retired schoolteacher. Betty did not realize that the slowing of estrogen production can result in sudden and serious depression. "There had been a lot of ups and downs in my life the year it started, including my retirement from teaching, and I thought I was simply a little blue.

"But my feelings of profound sorrowfulness got progressively worse, to the point where I didn't even want to get out of bed in the morning. Sometimes I felt so despondent I even considered suicide, though I never acted on those feelings. Finally, I decided to get a checkup."

Knowing that Betty was in the middle of menopause, I conducted a series of blood tests to check her estrogen levels and found that her ovaries had all but ceased production. I told Betty there was a good chance that her low estrogen level was compounding the sadness she felt as a result of the dramatic changes that her body was going through. Depression is fairly common in women of Betty's age.

I suggested that Betty try a regimen of low-dose estrogen supplements and the antidepressant Prozac, which has shown good results in cases such as this. She agreed, and was amazed at the resulting changes in her mood.

"The turnaround was startling," she said later. "Within a few weeks I felt almost completely normal again. I no longer burst into tears at the drop of a hat, nor did I dread getting out of bed in the morning."

Like your first menstrual period or the birth of your first child, the onset of menopause marks a new stage in a woman's life, creating new challenges that affect each woman differently. The fact that some women greet the onset of menopause with apprehension and anxiety has a lot to do with the amount of misinformation and superstition that surround a woman's change of life. Menopause does not signal "old age," nor is it an indication of increasingly poor health or a sexual crisis, though it may be misinterpreted that way by women who lack knowledge of what is going on inside their bodies during this physiological process. Even your health care provider may not be properly up to date on the subject or sensitive enough to your particular concerns.

The story of each woman's journey through

menopause is unique. Your experience will not be exactly the same as that of your best friend, mother, or sister, though there will be many shared traits. The nature and intensity of your own experience will determine what treatment options, if any, are right for you. At one end of the spectrum are women who seem to breeze through menopause with very few troublesome symptoms. They enjoy the absence of menstrual cycles and are glad that they do not have to worry about accidental pregnancy. Other women are less lucky. They may have several years of irregular periods, hot flashes that interfere with work and social activities, depression, painful intercourse, and a general dissatisfaction with their dryer skin and thinner hair. Most women fall somewhere in between, experiencing some discomfort or anxiety during one or more stages of menopause. This chapter aims to educate you about what to expect during this phase of your life and explain estrogen's role in the process.

Q: What does the word "menopause" mean?
A: It is derived from the Greek words "monthly" and "cause to cease," and means "to stop menstruating." That is exactly what happens, and doctors use it as one guideline in diagnosing menopause. But there is much more to menopause than that. For one thing, you do not stop menstruating suddenly. It is a gradual process with various stages and specific changes that take place at certain times. Understanding the process—having knowledge about what changes

are taking place in your body—can make a big difference in what kind of menopause experience you have both physically and emotionally.

Q: What's the first sign of menopause?
A: Usually it is just an irregularity in periods. Sometimes you miss one now and then. Sometimes they even come sooner than usual. This can go on for as long as four years. Many women have hot flashes during the same period.

Q: When do most women start menopause?
A: The average age is forty-six to fifty-six. But 1 percent of women undergo premature menopause before age forty. Few women realize that menopause is a process that begins several years before they notice any changes. Ovulation starts to decline between ages thirty-eight and forty-two. This starts a kind of domino effect: fewer eggs mean less estrogen, and this makes levels of FSH and LH increase, in order to compensate. When they get high enough, menopause is established.

Q: What are the different stages of menopause?
A: First is the early or "perimenopausal" stage, meaning "around the time of menopause." It may begin around age forty-five and is associated with the beginning of estrogen decline. This occurs at different rates for different women, so the symptoms vary widely. Some women start having hot flashes almost right away; most just have vague feelings of uneasiness or physical

discomfort, or have "odd periods." Few women realize this is how menopause begins. More of them associate menopause with the second stage, which is when periods become far less frequent and eventually stop all together. During this stage the ovaries finally cease producing estrogen. The postmenopausal period follows final cessation of menstruation. All of this can take an average of ten years.

Q: Which is the most troublesome part?
A: Physically, that varies from woman to woman. Emotionally, many women worry more at the beginning because they fear the worst. Many women do not find any part troublesome.

Q: What hormonal changes take place?
A: The cessation of ovulation results in the reduction of estrogen levels. There is also a change in the kind of estrogen; after menopause, you have lower levels of the more potent estradiol, which is made in the ovary, and higher levels of the weaker estrone, which is made in fat and other tissues. FSH levels go way up. Androstenedione, which is made in the ovary, is reduced by about half as ovarian activity declines. But testosterone hardly changes at all. That is significant because testosterone contributes to sexuality. It may be an androgen/estrogen imbalance that causes symptoms such as falling hair, excess facial hair, and oily skin.

Q: What physical changes happen when estrogen declines, and what symptoms do they cause?

A: The breasts become smaller and change shape, and fibrocystic problems diminish. The outer part of the cervix becomes thinner and more easily damaged. Menstrual irregularities occur. The blood supply to the uterus diminishes and it becomes smaller and less weighty. The vagina shortens and narrows and becomes less elastic, which can cause painful intercourse. The outside of the vulva gets thinner and weaker and is more easily injured or inflamed; it may itch or be painful during intercourse. Body fat may shift to a slightly different pattern. Lipid metabolism changes and calcium moves out of the bones, producing higher risks of heart disease and osteoporosis.

Q: Do women ever just suddenly stop menstruating completely?

A: Yes: women who have "surgical menopause" from removal of the ovaries, and about 10 percent of other women.

Q: I've heard menopause called "a disease," "a natural process," "the failure of the ovaries," and "a new beginning." Which is it?

A: Biologically speaking, it is quite simple. The ovaries are designed to do a particular job—produce eggs and the hormones needed to support pregnancy. When the biologically ideal time for a woman to have babies is over, the ovaries stop working at it. That is really all there is to it. The other terms all reflect a point of view.

Q: What does "climacteric" mean?
A: It is another word for menopause. But it is a particularly interesting term because it is derived from the Greek word meaning "a rung of a ladder," which is suggestive of "climbing up" or "moving on" rather than ending something.

Q: What causes hot flashes?
A: Declining estrogen levels are the root cause, but the immediate cause is that the body is trying to cool off. You are not really hotter—the temperature in the room, for example, is the same for you as for everybody else in it. But lack of estrogen makes your temperature regulator (the hypothalamus) unable to read temperature signals properly. Thus, a temperature that should be comfortable registers in your hypothalamus as too hot. To reduce the heat, blood moves toward the skin surface where some of the heat can "leak out" into the air. And that is what makes you suddenly flush with heat.

Q: What is a hot flash actually like?
A: Some people experience an aura—a disturbance in perception—the way people with migraine headaches do. It is a feeling of uneasiness, almost anxiety, as if something unpleasant is about to happen. Sometimes you might feel palpitations, or feel headachy or dizzy. This lasts no more than a minute. Then a sense of warmth

starts in your upper chest and moves up your neck and head, turning into intense heat as it occurs. You may perspire, and your heart may feel as if it is racing or palpating. Your skin reddens. Finally, after about five minutes, you perspire, which cools you off so that you may feel chilled.

Q: When during the day or night do women usually have hot flashes?
A: They are most frequent in the daytime, especially early in the day and toward late afternoon and early evening. They are less frequent at night but may be stronger.

Q: How long does each hot flash last?
A: It can be over in an instant or last for several minutes. Five minutes is a typical maximum, although you may feel somewhat uncomfortable for as long as half an hour after the flash itself is over.

Q: How many hot flashes do women have per day?
A: Some women do not even have one every day. Only about half of all women between age forty and sixty report daily hot flashes. Small minorities have more than one a day or fewer than one a week.

Q: How long—in months or years—do hot flashes go on?
A: First, remember that they do not continue at the same rate; women may have them for as long as five years but after the first year or two, they

become less and less frequent. Women who are active in taking care of their health usually find ways of relieving their hot flashes fairly early in menopause, so no matter how long they last, they are not as troublesome.

Q: Besides hot flashes, what symptoms do women complain of most?
A: That is an interesting question, because there is a difference between what symptoms women have most often and what symptoms bother them the most. Physically, hot flashes and vaginal dryness are the two symptoms experienced most often by women who have symptoms at all, and they may be the ones that bother a woman most. But other symptoms may be first on some women's lists of complaints. For example, irritability is a problem some women would like to get rid of. Another is insomnia. It is important to remember that the basic changes in menopause are much the same for everybody, but women are very individual in their feelings, symptoms, and reactions.

Q: Does estrogen decline always cause depression?
A: There is a tremendous difference of opinion whether decreased estrogen levels *ever* cause depression. Nobody has ever done a scientific study that proves a connection. It is important not to confuse mood swings or emotional unease with depression. Estrogen does seem to have a lot to do with the emotional ups and downs of menopause, because of the connection between

estrogen and the hypothalamus, which helps regulate mood. But depression is a specific diagnosis not attributable to menopause itself and actually more likely to affect younger women. Some women get depressed—or perhaps to be more exact, sorrowful—around menopause, but there are many possible reasons for this. Menopause comes at a time when many things may happen to cause worry or sorrow: an important shift in your own or your husband's career or earning power, having to care for aging parents, adult children having money or marital problems, or fear of aging, which some people associate with menopause.

Q: **Lots of women say their mood gets better when they take hormones, so doesn't that mean that lack of hormones causes low moods?**

A: It is true that as the endocrine system becomes unstable so moods do, too. But women who report improved mood after hormone therapy may just be feeling much better because they are not having hot flashes, they are sleeping better, and they are cheered up because their skin and hair look healthier.

Q: **Do alcohol and cigarettes affect menopause symptoms?**

A: Smoking reduces estrogen levels so smokers tend to have earlier menopause. Smoking and excessive alcohol use are important factors in the risk of postmenopausal osteoporosis.

Q: Why do I wake up with wet sheets, when I rarely sweat much during the day, even when I am having hot flashes?

A: One reason is that night hot flashes are often more intense. Equally important is that at night you are covered by blankets or even in the summertime by at least a sheet. This prevents the heat from escaping into the air as it does in the daytime, and it also prevents your perspiration from evaporating, which would otherwise help you cool down. You may want to anticipate this and use lighter or more open-weave, natural fiber covers. All-cotton sheets are much better than cotton-polyester combinations. Many women solve the problem by sleeping in a colder room—opening windows in winter or using air conditioning in summer.

Q: What makes me sometimes wake up in the night shivering?

A: After a hot flash and a night sweat, lying in a damp bed eventually brings your body temperature way down.

Q: Lately I've been finding I just can't stand having my husband in the same bed while I sleep because he's so warm. What can I do?

A: First, assuming that your discomfort is due to your temperature-regulating problem, you may want to talk to your doctor about medical treatment for the hot flashes. But you also should have an open discussion with your husband, explaining the purely physical nature of the difficulty. Keep in mind that with your elevated temperature and perhaps night sweats, he may be having some discomfort, too. You should be able to work out some solution; the problem is not permanent.

Q: **Why am I having hot flashes *during* menstruation, right at the beginning? I do not have them any other time.**

A: Sometimes, especially early in menopause when some estrogen is still being produced, a woman's estrogen and FSH levels will be menopausal only at certain times (say, in early menstruation) and normal at all other times. There also may be other causes of hot flashes, which your doctor needs to determine. They include hyperthyroidism (an overactive thyroid gland), alcoholism, and diabetes.

Q: **Do certain things trigger hot flashes?**

A: Yes, but they vary with individuals so you need to learn which ones may affect you. Stress is a common trigger; so are caffeine, alcohol, hot foods and drinks, sugar, spices, hot rooms, or hot beds.

Q: **I'm not being seriously troubled by menopausal symptoms, but I just don't like the way I look, and I'm not even sure why. Any suggestions?**

A: Since estrogen is essential for healthy skin, when the levels are lowered the skin seems to lose some of its tone. It may be drier than it was, which makes it lose its glow. Aside from HRT, you can use neutral, nondrying, nonallergenic soap, rinse thoroughly, and use a good moisturizer that is not oily.

Q: How often should I see my gynecologist during menopause?
A: Your gynecologist will establish a schedule if you are having symptoms or being treated for them. You may also see an endocrinologist on occasion. In addition, you should continue—or finally start—routine checkups for specific tests: a Pap smear annually, and a mammogram every one or two years between ages forty and fifty and every year after fifty. Your own physician should recommend any other routine tests specifically appropriate for you, such as thyroid function tests or bone density measurements.

Q: My doctor said it's harder to do a Pap smear now that I've been through menopause. Why is that?
A: With menopause and age the cervix shrinks and tends to withdraw up into the vagina or become flush with the vaginal wall. This simply makes it a little harder to find in order to do the slight scraping needed to get cells for the test. But it can—and should—still be done.

Q: After menopause, your ovaries are useless, so why not have them removed to prevent ovarian cancer?
A: Some specialists do recommend it. Ovarian cancer is especially dangerous because it produces few or no early symptoms and thus is

rarely diagnosed until it reaches the later, harder-to-treat stages. But this is a matter of individual choice, influenced by a number of significant factors: Do you have a family history that puts you at high risk for ovarian cancer? If not, is it worth the risks of surgery just to ease your mind, considering that ovarian cancer is not that common? But other physicians say healthy ovaries should never be removed, either before or after menopause. You should be well informed and discuss this with medical specialists, counselors, and family members before making a decision.

Q: I'm pretty sure I'm starting menopause, but the doctor said that age forty is too young and my symptoms are probably just due to stress. Who's right?

A: You certainly could be. Although forty is at the very low end of the age range, it is not impossible, and some women have started menopause even earlier. In fact, as many as 5 percent of the women in this country under the age of thirty-five undergo early menopause. But doctors do not consider that to be menopause and term it "premature ovarian failure." Most endocrinologists and gynecologists feel strongly that such women should be considered high-priority candidates for treatment, especially if they still want to have children. It is important for women in that age range to see their doctors promptly if they experience what seem to be menopausal symptoms, while it is still early enough to perhaps maintain egg production.

Q: Is there a test for menopause?

A: Not really. Low levels of estrogen and high levels of FSH are indicators that menopause is underway. But it can be absolutely diagnosed only after it is over—some doctors say after no menstrual periods have occurred for six months, others say for a year, with no pregnancy or other condition to account for the absence of periods.

Q: Why do women in the menopausal years always seem to gain weight in the upper body?

A: Although some women do gain weight during the menopausal and postmenopausal years, what you are talking about may not be weight gain so much as weight redistribution. At puberty, when estrogen begins to make its impact, body fat shifts to the more female pattern, emphasizing hips and buttocks. With menopause and estrogen depletion, the pattern sometimes shifts back somewhat, with fat being reduced around the hips and increased at the waist and above. Not all women experience this change, and your basic body type makes a difference.

Q: Why do some women have much worse hot flashes than others?

A: There is a definite connection between the amount of decline in estrogen levels. That is the primary reason. It may also be that the interplay between estrogen, the hypothalamus, and the nervous system—which work together to control temperature—is more sensitive or more easily disrupted in some women than in others.

Q: Am I imagining things, or are my breasts getting less lumpy than they were before menopause?
A: It is quite common for women who tend to have fibrocystic or lumpy breasts to notice this change. It is part of the general shrinkage and reshaping of the breast that accompanies lower estrogen.

Q: What's going to happen to my sex life?
A: That is entirely up to you and your partner. Nothing happens biologically or hormonally to prevent or alter sexual activity except those changes that can make intercourse uncomfortable—and they can be prevented or treated. For example, you could try using vaginal lubricants, having intercourse often, changing both the type and amount of foreplay, or using HRT, or alternative treatments. Some women find sex more pleasurable after menopause because there is no possibility of pregnancy. Whether libido decreases with menopause or because of menopause is a highly controversial issue. Some people say it declines, others that it never changes. Older people may become more inhibited because they have the idea that for them to have sex is somehow taboo or even offensive to others. These and many other issues are involved in women's sexual lives with regard to menopause and advancing age. There is a wealth of information, help, and counseling available. But remember that there is nothing physically or biologically inherent in menopause that would significantly interfere with a healthy sex life.

Q: Are there particular urinary problems during menopause?

A: The most common is incontinence, or leaking of urine, which can be of two kinds. One is called stress incontinence, which means urine escapes when you cough, laugh, or strain yourself lifting, so that the abdomen presses on the bladder. The other is called urge incontinence, which means that when you have the urge to urinate, you cannot control it for as long as you once could. A major factor is the loss of muscle tone in the bladder and the pelvis. Estrogen does contribute to the condition of these muscles, so its decline could affect bladder control. But it is somewhat difficult to separate the influence of menopause from that of age, which obviously contributes. Whatever the reason, one effective solution is to ask your doctor for instruction in exercises that can improve the condition of the critical muscles. Another problem is that the thinning of tissues in the urinary tract makes the urinary tract more susceptible to infection. If you feel as if you have to urinate too often, if you feel greater urgency when your bladder is full, or if you have burning on urination, consult your doctor, who can diagnose and treat infections—and also determine if the cause is not infection but vaginal irritation.

Q: Recently my eyes seem very sensitive, and wearing contact lenses is becoming uncomfortable. Is it true that this is due to menopause?

A: Dry eye syndrome, or *keratoconjunctivitis sicca*, is common during menopause, as well as during menstruation or contraceptive use among young women who wear contact lenses. Symptoms include red eyelids, temporary vision problems, and sudden unexplained tears. It is believed that the cycling of reproductive hormones has something to do with this problem. But, surprisingly little is understood about the association between "dry eye" and menopause. The symptoms do seem to be linked to low levels of both estrogen and progesterone, so if you are considering hormone therapy, you would probably do better with combined hormones than estrogen replacement alone. You should make sure your eye specialist knows that you are menopausal.

Q: I haven't had a period for so long that I thought I was finished with menopause. But this week I had some bleeding. Is this normal?

A: There is not any real "normal" in regard to menstrual patterns during the ten-year or so duration of menopause. Most women have irregular periods at the beginning, then they have very short menstrual periods spaced far apart, and finally no periods. But none of this is regular or predictable. The problem is that hormonal ups and downs during menopause—and the resulting irregular periods—depend on what is happening in the egg follicles and how that affects estrogen and FSH. But the activity in the follicles can be unpredictable. That is probably the explanation for your unexpected bleeding, but you should certainly discuss it with your gynecologist to be sure there is no other reason for it, especially if you are experiencing bleeding one year after you have stopped menstruating.

Q: Does menopause make hair fall out?
A: Some women notice an increase in hair loss during menopause, which is related to decline in estrogen. In fact, sometimes this occurs early, even before menstrual irregularity or hot flashes. It is not usually serious, and it can be restored with hormone therapy. Younger women with hair loss who are highly unlikely to be menopausal may be suffering a related problem—an excess of androgens; this can also be treated.

Q: If I'm still having a period about every three or four months, with no regular pattern, can I get pregnant?
A: Yes. What is also significant is that because of the irregularity, you might not realize that you are pregnant until the pregnancy is somewhat advanced. If you do not want to be pregnant, you should continue to use a birth control method. Your doctor can inform you when menopause is completely established, usually about a year after your last period. You should discuss with your gynecologist at that time whether or not contraceptive pills are still advisable.

Q: Why does the skin start to sag around menopause?
A: Sagging is one of several skin changes, including drying and thinning. An important component in skin is collagen, a form of connective

tissue related to bone and cartilage. It consists of tough, nonstretchy fibers that make the skin firm and give it support. Low levels of estrogen result in a decrease in collagen; thus, the skin simply loses its internal support. The same thing happens in the vagina and uterus, sometimes with serious results. With enough collagen loss, these structures may sag sufficiently to cause part of the bladder, uterus, or rectum to protrude into the vagina. The result may be urine leakage when you cough, sneeze, or strain, and sometimes difficulty having a bowel movement. This is not common. It is even less of a problem among women receiving hormone therapy.

Q: When do women become susceptible to osteoporosis: before, during, or after menopause?
A: The breaking down and building up of bone is a lifelong process, but at a certain point, the breakdown exceeds the buildup, and bones become hollow and brittle. Both men and women undergo this breakdown with age, but with women the process begins much earlier and is more pronounced. Women begin to lose bone mass at a small but significant rate when they are in their forties, whether they are undergoing menopause or not. But, the loss of bone speeds up as estrogen levels decrease during menopause and afterwards. Most women get inadequate calcium in their diets throughout their lives, and women approaching menopause often suffer a definite shortage. (See Chapter 4, "Osteoporosis.")

Q: Right after I started having hot flashes, I developed carpal tunnel syndrome. Is there a connection?

A: Carpal tunnel syndrome, which involves compression of a nerve in your wrist or hand, is sometimes included in lists of menopausal effects, but there may or may not be a connection in any individual case. The immediate cause of the problem is repetitive damaging motions—typing, using a computer, twisting motions such as using a wrench or screwdriver—so you need to identify what you are doing to trigger the condition. At menstrual age, you may be more susceptible because estrogen loss weakens connective tissue, but it could also be due to early rheumatoid arthritis. Not everything that happens during menopause is caused by menopause.

Q: I've suffered from mild to moderately severe depression much of my life. Is menopause going to make it worse?

A: There is no way of knowing. Being convinced you are going to be depressed could cause it to happen. Since you have this concern, you should consider discussing it with your physician and your therapist, and perhaps there might be consultation between the two, so that they could suggest a plan that might include hormone therapy, an antidepressant, or possibly hormone replacement with counseling or psychotherapy. Much of the depression associated with menopause has to do with feeling physically bad, so perhaps all you need is relief from symptoms.

Q: Why do the ovaries keep producing testosterone after menopause?
A: It appears to be nature's way of trying to keep the endocrine system in some sort of balance. When estrogen declines, testosterone and androstenedione are converted into estrogen by body fat. In fact, they are the source of most of the estrogen in your body after menopause.

Q: I had my first period rather late, at fourteen. Does that mean my menopause will also start late?
A: Not necessarily. It is not considered late to have your first period at age fourteen. It is less usual to start menstruating at age fifteen or sixteen; this may be due to low levels of gonadotropin or a problem with ovarian function. (By contrast, some young women begin menstruating at eight or even earlier, due to premature release of gonadotropin.) It is hard to predict when you will start menopause, unless you can detect a pattern among your female relatives who have already started or gone through menopause.

Q: I've heard that when I start menopause I may have oily skin and extra facial hair just as I did when I first started menstruating. Is that true?
A: No. Quite the reverse. Those symptoms— along with the growth of pubic hair and the onset of underarm hair and odor—are caused by

excess androgen. During puberty, the body is just starting to produce these hormones along with estrogen, and the balance is not always quite right.

Q: It seems to me that my friends who are thin complain more about menopause than the ones who are overweight. If so, why should that be?

A: Menopausal symptoms are due to estrogen and progesterone depletion that occurs when the ovaries stop producing eggs. But fat tissue is also able to produce estrogen, sometimes enough to counteract the ovarian decline at least partially. Some other tissues and glands also contribute, but to a much smaller extent.

Q: What's the difference between natural menopause and menopause brought on by surgery or cancer treatment?

A: Both, of course, result in a decrease in estrogen levels, but removing the ovaries or chemically stopping them from functioning makes the drop sudden and dramatic, and the symptoms are equally sudden and dramatic. Women tend to be both physically and psychologically somewhat prepared for menopause when it happens naturally because it is gradual. Only about one in ten women going through natural menopause stop menstruating abruptly. With "artificial" menopause, it is always sudden and dramatic, so the adjustment may be much harder.

Q: What makes intercourse so uncomfortable after menopause?

A: Another way of looking at it is to ask why intercourse is comfortable before menopause. Estrogen's natural role is to keep the outer lining of the vulva thick and resistant to damage and to trigger production of lubricants when needed. With menopause, there often is too little estrogen in circulation to do all of its usual jobs as well as usual.

Q: Do women who have never been pregnant undergo menopause at a different age than those who have?

A: Not necessarily. The endocrine system seems to "wind down" egg production after a certain time as if it were triggered by the total number of eggs that have been released, not by how many were fertilized.

THREE

⁓✸⁓

Heart Disease

CASE STUDY

Women often have to fight harder than men for equal care when a heart attack occurs. Jennifer, a 58-year-old airline ticketing agent, found this out when she experienced sudden chest pains and was rushed to the hospital by her husband. Tests revealed that she had suffered a mild heart attack as a result of coronary artery disease and that she was probably at risk for another heart attack if she did not receive treatment. She is well read and current in her knowledge of health care, so she was not surprised when her cardiologist broke the news to her.

"What did surprise me," she said later, "was that he didn't recommend an evaluation for angioplasty or a similar procedure as a preventive measure. I'm no doctor, but it seemed like the logical thing to do. When my father had a heart attack, his doctor insisted on angioplasty as soon as he was well enough."

Jennifer brought up the issue a couple of days later, and was shocked and angered by her doctor's response. "He told me that women my age typically don't have serious heart attacks, and that I would probably be fine if I just watched my diet and exercised more. He also suggested I look into hormone replacement therapy if I wasn't already receiving it. That's all he told me."

As soon as Jennifer checked out of the hospital, she went to another heart specialist with her concerns. He performed a series of tests that confirmed that three of her coronary arteries were dangerously blocked, and suggested angioplasty as soon as possible. Jennifer underwent the potentially life-saving procedure one week later and has felt fine ever since.

"I still get angry when I think about my stay in the hospital," Jennifer says. "I received less-than-adequate health care advice simply because I was a woman. If it had been my husband in that hospital bed, the cardiologist almost certainly would have recommended angioplasty without thinking twice."

CASE STUDY

When 52-year-old Teresa's mother died from a heart attack at age seventy-two, Teresa wasted no time in changing her lifestyle to insure that she would not suffer a similar fate. "My mother and I were alike in many ways, and I wanted to make sure I wasn't going to be a victim of my family's lousy health history," she told me. "I talked at length with my family physician and he told me that while heart attacks were more common in men than women, there was a strong likelihood that I was at risk for heart disease sometime in my life. That scared me."

Teresa, a pastry chef, followed her doctor's advice and literally turned her life around. She started eating better, began exercising regularly, reduced her alcohol intake, and stopped smoking immediately. So when she came to me at the onset of menopause, I suggested hormone replacement therapy (HRT) as a way of both easing her menopause symptoms and further reducing her risk of heart disease.

"Heart disease has always been my primary concern," Teresa says. "I sleep better at night knowing HRT is reducing my risk while helping me cope with menopause."

Most women that I treat are far more afraid of breast cancer than of heart attacks, and even national health organizations tend to give more publicity to the dangers of breast cancer over those of heart disease in women. Yet heart attacks kill a quarter of a million women every year—five times the mortality rate of breast cancer. Many women are not even aware of their level of heart-disease risk. Although heart disease has been a major killer of women for a great many years, virtually no significant scientific research on heart disease in women had been conducted until very recently. Many physicians have not had the information necessary to make valid recommendations about heart health to their female patients.

The most important basic fact is that the risk of heart disease for women changes dramatically over a lifetime. Women do have one advantage over men: Before menopause, few women suffer from heart disease compared with men, and even after menopause, they tend to have heart attacks much later in life. The advantage begins to shrink after age fifty, and at age sixty the risk is almost exactly the same as a man's. After age seventy-five, a woman's risk is greater than a man's.

In the early years of hormone therapy for menopause, it was thought that estrogen given alone reduced the dangers of heart disease and osteoporosis, but probably increased the risk of uterine cancer; however, this link was never proven conclusively. Estrogen replacement therapy (ERT) thus achieved a negative image among women, even though it improved their survival rate overall because of its significant effect on reducing the risk of heart attack. Some women have now become concerned about recent reports that the hormone progestin, often used in combination with estrogen, nullifies estrogen's protective effect on the heart. As of yet, this nullifying effect has not yet been established, and preliminary evidence suggests that the reports may be inaccurate. (See Chapter 6, "Risks and Myths.")

Q: What type of heart disease is most common in women?

A: When anyone talks about heart disease as a life-threatening illness, it is almost always in reference to coronary artery disease. This results from the clogging or narrowing of blood vessels that supply the heart with blood. The narrowing is caused by atherosclerosis (fatty hardening), also known as arteriosclerosis. When deprived of adequate oxygen, the heart cannot pump effectively and the lungs do not get enough oxygen. Shortness of breath or chest pain (angina pectoris) may be experienced.

Heart attack or myocardial infarction (heart muscle destruction) results when this oxygen deprivation is so overwhelming that areas of heart muscle die, making those parts of the heart unable to continue pumping. Occasionally, the result is an uncoordinated, weak rhythm that can be fatal within moments.

A less dramatic but also dangerous condition, congestive heart failure, results when the heart is still pumping, but weakly. Fluid backs up in the lungs and interferes with normal breathing and oxygen transfer.

Q: Is it true that heart attacks in women are worse than in men?

A: This question does not have a simple answer. There are some facts that shed a little light on the issue. One study, reported in the *Journal of Women's Health*, revealed that women who have had a heart attack and heart surgery suffer more postoperative psychological symptoms than men; these symptoms include depression, fear of resuming sexual activity, and unhealthy haste to return to family duties. In spite of this, women are often not referred to postsurgery rehabilitation programs, and when they are, their attendance is not as good as men's. It is not easy to account for these findings. Regardless of the seriousness of the heart attack, women are more physically ill afterward than men are. One large study, reported in the prestigious *New England Journal of Medicine*, identified one reason for this: Doctors do not act as aggressively to intervene in ways that might prevent the progression of heart disease among women as they do with men. As an example, among one group of people whose stress tests indicated a heart problem, 40 percent of men but only 4 percent of women were then referred for an angiogram, which is a diagnostic test that reveals blocking of arteries. The *Journal* named this "the Yentl syndrome," after the woman in the Isaac Bashevis Singer story (and Barbra Streisand movie) who had to disguise herself as a man in order to study Jewish law. Finally, perhaps because coronary heart disease is not as common among women under fifty as it is among men the same age, physicians are less likely to be concerned about chest pains or other danger signs of potential heart disease in women of this age as they are in male patients.

The medical profession is beginning to take notice of and concern itself with research and treatment of heart disease among women. But it is still very much a woman's responsibility to be alert to heart disease risks or symptoms, to take the initiative in reducing her own risks, and to make sure her physician is equally involved.

Q: What makes someone more at risk for heart disease?

A: There are a number of known factors. First, genetics: If your mother or father died of a heart attack before age sixty, your risk is considerably escalated. Second, gender: Men have more than three times the risk of developing heart disease than women—until menopause erases the female advantage. Third, the presence of either diabetes mellitus or a family history of diabetes makes a woman's risk level about the same as that of a man's, even before menopause. High blood pressure, high cholesterol levels, and obesity (particularly when associated with other illnesses and with elevated cholesterol) are important influences. Chronic stress—from emotional, family, or work problems—is another factor. The most dramatic risk factor—and one that you can do something about (unlike genetics)—is smoking. It is the most important risk factor for women under forty and is a considerable factor for those over forty. Finally, of course, is the increased risk that follows menopause. The difference is particularly striking among women who have undergone menopause at an earlier-than-usual age, either through surgery, chemotherapy for cancer, or premature ovarian failure.

Q: What is cholesterol and how is it different from saturated fat?

A: Cholesterol is a natural fatty substance that is made in the body and is also found in food such as egg yolks, various oils, animal fat, and organ meats (liver, kidneys). Elevated cholesterol is an important heart disease risk factor. In general, a cholesterol level of less than 200 mg/dl is considered okay, 200 to 239 is borderline risky, and 240 is high. It is also important to remember that people whose cholesterol level is considered only borderline may have varying degrees of risk. Borderline high cholesterol is not much of a risk factor for people with no other factors, but it is more serious if, for example, you have a family history of heart disease, if you smoke, or if you have low LDL, diabetes, or severe obesity. Anyone with borderline cholesterol should try to reduce it through dietary changes and should have their cholesterol level checked at least once a year. Those with borderline cholesterol plus other risk factors should begin a stringent dietary control program and have their cholesterol checked frequently, with medication as a possible option if diet does not work.

Saturated fat, found in meats, eggs, dairy products, and certain oils, is readily converted into cholesterol in the body. Polyunsaturated fats (such as corn oil) tend to reduce cholesterol, and monounsaturated fats (such as olive oil) have no effect either way.

Although cholesterol is essential to life (it is the necessary foundation for all of the steroid hormones including sex hormones), it is not necessary to eat cholesterol-containing foods. After infancy, the body manufactures cholesterol from internal sources.

Q: What's the significance of LDL and HDL?
A: Both are lipoproteins, meaning they are proteins that transport fat in the bloodstream. Low-density lipoprotein (LDL) tends to carry fat right to the artery walls and unload it. The fat remains there unless it is removed by high-density lipoprotein (HDL) and transferred to the liver, which either breaks it down and gets rid of it or uses it to make bile salts. Popularly, HDL is known as "good" cholesterol and LDL as "bad" cholesterol. The more HDL you have, the better your cardiovascular health is likely to be.

Q: How much LDL should I have at age fifty-five?
A: That is hard to say without knowing more about you. Recent guidelines say that you can have as much as 130 mg/dl of LDL if you have no family history of heart disease or any other risk factors. With risk factors, your LDL level should be 100 mg/dl; many physicians recommend this level regardless of risk.

What is probably more important for women is the proportion of HDL to LDL. The reason is that estrogen boosts HDL, which probably accounts a great deal for premenopausal women's lower risk of heart disease compared with that of men. When estrogen declines after menopause, HDL may also decline, reducing your protection against the negative effects of LDLs. Other factors associated with lower HDL are elevated testosterone and obesity. Total cholesterol in relation to HDL and LDL is also significant. All of these need to be carefully weighed by a knowledgeable physician in assessing your cardiovascular risk and making recommendations regarding HRT.

Q: **In spite of drastic changes in my diet and exercise habits, my total cholesterol and my LDL cholesterol are still dangerously high. Is there anything else I can do?**

A: If the term "dangerous" has been applied to your cholesterol and LDL levels by a doctor or on the basis of repeated blood analysis (because an isolated test can be misleading), then you may want to discuss your diet with someone especially knowledgeable about nutrition and heart disease. "Drastic" changes can sometimes be as unhealthy as no change at all. If you adopt a sensible weight-loss and cholesterol-reduction plan (that includes both nutrition and exercise) and stick to it for a while but still see no improvement, then you just may be one of those people who are physiologically resistant to such measures. You may want to discuss with your doctor the possibility of your taking a similar prescription medication that can lower your LDL and reduce your risk. If you are postmenopausal, HRT is also a potentially effective option.

Q: I've heard that "women who work like men have heart attacks like men." Is that true?

A: Not necessarily. In fact, work per se, even hard work or high-pressure work, is not an important risk factor. What does matter is the kind of work you do. It is been demonstrated that working at jobs that are very demanding but not very rewarding does contribute to high blood pressure and other health problems among men— so presumably this would be also true of women. The problem is that women tend to work at such jobs in far greater numbers than men; that is, waiting tables, routine computer inputting, or doing clerical and other "support" tasks that do not involve much decision-making, creativity, or recognition and reward. The well-known Framingham Heart Study, which has provided so much of the information on heart disease in both men and women, showed that women clerical workers have more heart attacks than women with domestic responsibilities.

Q: What can be done to reduce the risk of heart attack?

A: Quitting smoking is the best thing you can do for yourself, not just to reduce heart disease risk but to reduce the risk of lethal lung diseases and various other illnesses—not to mention looking and feeling vastly better. Within three or four years of quitting, your risk of heart disease drops down to where it would be if you had never smoked.

You cannot change your genes, of course, but

you can offset heredity to a considerable extent by taking all the other steps to reduce your overall risk. It is extremely important to have regular medical checkups and get treatment for conditions such as diabetes and high blood pressure. Weight control, reduction of cholesterol, and an appropriate exercise program are all recommended for improving your heart disease risk. Hormone replacement is an option that is strongly recommended for women with greater-than-average risk, for example, those with an unfavorable lipid profile or a family history of heart disease.

Some preliminary results from a new study at the Washington University School of Medicine in St. Louis suggest that a combination of vigorous exercise and HRT has a better effect on your lipid profiles than either alone. The scientists there studied seventy-one women between sixty and seventy-two years old. Some were treated with exercise alone, some with HRT alone, and some with exercise and HRT combined; some women were not treated at all so they could serve as controls for comparison. The women in the exercise groups started out at low intensity for two months and switched to vigorous workouts for the next nine months. At the end of the eleven months, the women in the exercise-only group had lower levels of total cholesterol and low-density lipoproteins (LDLs), but their levels of high-density lipoproteins (HDLs) did not change. HRT subjects had lower LDLs and higher HDLs but no change in total cholesterol.

The HRT plus exercise group had lower total cholesterol and LDLs and higher HDLs.

Q: What is the link between diabetes and heart attack?

A: A diabetic has higher blood pressure and higher insulin levels which increase cardiac risk. The current understanding is that high blood-sugar levels somehow change the condition of the artery walls so that they are more susceptible to narrowing by deposits of fat.

Q: Does aspirin help prevent heart attacks in women as it does in men?

A: This is another one of those issues regarding women's heart health where the information is not as complete as it is for men. Studies of aspirin use in women have only recently begun, while those in men have been going on for many years. A study of ninety thousand women nurses indicated that taking one to six aspirins a week reduced the heart attack risk by 30 percent, compared to a 50 percent reduction of risk among men in similar studies. The difference may be due to the men's far stricter and more carefully controlled schedule of treatment compared with that of the women, as opposed to aspirin being less effective in women. Another study of men and women who were already known to have heart disease showed that taking half a baby aspirin a day reduced the risk of heart attack for both sexes. Despite these encouraging results, you should not make the decision to take aspirin as a preventive measure against heart attack without first consulting a specialist. Contrary to popular belief, aspirin use can carry some risks; you should be sure it poses no dangers to you.

Q: Why does menopause increase women's risk of heart attack?

A: It is assumed that premenopausally, estrogen protects against heart disease, and that the post-menopausal decline in natural estrogen production removes that protection. This stands to reason, since the most dramatic change in menopause, and the apparent cause of menopausal symptoms, is estrogen deprivation. What is not so obvious is exactly how estrogen works to protect against heart disease.

Some details are known. First, there are estrogen receptors in the arteries; that is, cells designed so that estrogen can attach to them. Such receptor cells in the body almost always mean that some significant action takes place between the substance and the receptor. It is not known exactly what the action is, but there are several clues to the meaning of the receptors, as well as other possible direct effects of estrogen: it may enhance the effectiveness of the healthier fats in the bloodstream; it might block the constricting effect of certain chemicals; it could increase the activity of prostacyclin, which has a beneficial effect on vessel health; it could directly prevent the fatty deposits in the vessel walls; or it might inhibit deposits on vessel walls by increasing blood flow. Relating to this last point, studies have shown that the slowing of blood flow after menopause can be improved by 50 percent with just six weeks of treatment with an estrogen patch.

Second, before menopause women have fewer red blood cells—and thus less iron—because of menstruation. Since men with high serum levels of iron have higher heart disease rates than those who do not, there appears to be a connection between menstruation, low iron, and low heart disease rates.

Finally, rates of death due to heart attacks have been shown to be lower among postmenopausal women taking estrogen compared with those not taking it.

Q: **Why is that so many things I read about estrogen and heart disease seem to contradict something else I just read the day before?**

A: Unfortunately, scientific knowledge about heart disease risks and estrogen is not as advanced as everybody would wish. Women's heart health has been neglected for many years while scientific researchers concentrated on what was thought to be of more critical concern, namely, men's heart disease risk. As a result, there may be two scientific studies on some specific topic—for example, whether estrogen increases or decreases the risk of blood clots—that differ dramatically from each other; it is impossible to decide which is correct because neither is absolutely conclusive. Many such studies are simply indicators of a need for more research in that particular topic, or are hints that there may be a problem in a particular area that should be taken into account when making decisions about treatments.

A good example is a study that shows that increased coronary heart disease risk among postmenopausal women is associated with higher levels of fibrinogen (a clotting factor) in the bloodstream. Higher fibrinogen in turn seems to be related to several factors, either alone or in combination, including increasing age, obesity, current cigarette smoking, moderate alcohol consumption, and a history of previous HRT. What does this mean? It is hard to say without knowing certain critical details, for example: What kind of previous HRT did the women have? Was it just for a few months for menopausal symptoms (if so, it would not be expected to improve heart disease risk factors)? Did they take estrogen alone or estrogen with progestin, and at what dosage levels?

Even the scientists who conducted this study said that it did not prove that higher fibrinogen levels actually increased risk. All that could be concluded at this stage is that if a woman has higher fibrinogen levels, it is a red flag signaling that she has some significant heart disease risk factors.

Q: If estrogen is so protective against heart attacks, why don't they give it to men?

A: In fact, there was an experiment some years ago in which men who had suffered heart attacks at an early age (before forty) were given estrogen in addition to the usual post–heart-attack treatment. They had a much lower rate of second heart attack and lower mortality than a comparable group of men who received conventional treatment alone, without estrogen. Unfortunately, the estrogen had the feminizing effects that would be expected: The men's breasts became enlarged, they developed fatty hips, and their voices became higher. These are side effects few men would be willing to live with regardless of any possible protective effects from the estrogen. Most people prefer to take chances on a future risk rather than suffer severe side effects in the present.

Q: How much difference in heart disease risk does estrogen actually make?

A: The answer varies depending on the kind of scientific study used for making an estimate. For example, the well-known Nurses' Health Study, which followed 48,470 postmenopausal nurses for ten years, found that estrogen-treated women had half the heart disease risk of untreated women. Another study, in which the women were all older than those in the nurses' survey, showed that the mortality rate for women who had taken estrogen at some time was 20 percent lower than for those who had never received estrogen treatment, and the rate among those who were taking estrogen at the time of the study was 40 percent lower. Most of this difference was due to differences in heart disease rates. A dramatic study of women who had been diagnosed as

having severe coronary artery disease showed
that the ten-year survival rate was 97 percent in
those taking estrogen compared with 60 percent
in untreated women. Whatever the actual numbers are, every study has shown that estrogen
reduces heart disease risk.

In an editorial in the *Journal of the American
Medical Association*, Dr. Bernadine Healy, former
director of the National Institutes of Health,
summed it up this way: "After a half century of
conflicting data, we can affirm with growing confidence that, at the very least, estrogen reduces
key cardiovascular risk factors in women at a
time when they become especially vulnerable to
heart disease, namely, after fifty years of age."

**Q: Does adding progestin to avoid endometrial risk
cancel out the good effect of estrogen on heart
disease risk?**
A: This was certainly a major concern when the
decision to add progestin was being weighed by
the medical profession. Theoretically, adding the
"male" hormone would put a woman right back
into the male risk status. But the progestin in
postmenopausal HRT is a low dose and is only
added for about twelve days a month, which
mimics the natural premenopausal pattern of
progesterone production. Thus, its effect on lipoproteins is considerably limited.

A very recent follow-up analysis of the Nurses'
Health Study showed that the risk of heart attack
was reduced by 40 percent in women who were
taking estrogen alone and by 61 percent in those

taking a combination of estrogen and progestin. The National Institutes of Health issued a caution about these findings, commenting that they are not "definite proof" that combination pills are better. The study, they said, just was not large enough or long enough. A positive conclusion probably cannot be reached until the conclusion of a major research project started in 1993 to examine specifically the relative merits of ERT and combined estrogen-progestin HRT.

Q: **Do all postmenopausal women have the same risk of heart disease?**
A: Not any more than all premenopausal women do. Let us assume, on a scale of one to ten, you have a heart disease risk of three and another woman has a risk of seven. After menopause, your risk may go up to five and hers may go up to ten. Your risk is worse than it was but is still better than hers.

Q: **What does "upper body overweight" mean?**
A: This term refers to a particular pattern of weight distribution that is significant in weighing heart disease risk—and that is related to hormones. There are three recognizable patterns of overweight. You may carry your extra pounds evenly over your whole body, which is common and has only a moderate influence on heart disease unless you are severely obese. Or you may have relatively slender legs, thighs, hips, and buttocks but a rounded abdomen and heavier bosom, upper back, and shoulders. This is called

upper body overweight. Or you may have a slender waist, bosom, and abdomen but heavy thighs, hips and buttocks. This is lower body overweight. Upper body (or upper segment) overweight is associated with higher risk factors for heart disease. This does not mean that of itself it puts you in more danger. It is instead a signal that your ovaries have always tended to produce a larger proportion of androgens ("male" hormones) than heart-protecting estrogen. This also means that you are more susceptible to diabetes or high blood pressure, which are also risk factors. Finally, fat from the abdomen is more easily carried by the bloodstream into the liver and thus is more easily translated into an unfavorable lipid profile.

Although people are "locked into" their body type early in life, that does not mean you cannot do anything about it. If you have upper body overweight, you should simply be more active in taking risk-reducing steps.

Q: Does heart disease risk go up as soon as menopause occurs?

A: No. It changes gradually over time; at the moment, there are no clear statistics about relative risk in the first year after menopause compared to, say, five years later. What is known is that between sixty and seventy, a woman's heart disease risk becomes about the same as a man's of the same age.

Q: Does it matter which kind of estrogen I take?
A: As far as the effect on the lipids and lipoproteins in your blood is concerned, there does seem to be a difference not only in the kind of estrogen you take but in the way in which you take it. The "natural" estrogens (those made in the laboratory to mimic the action of your own estrogen) seem to be less powerful than conjugated equine estrogen (from horses). Equine-derived estrogen not only works better than natural estrogen, it has no negative effects on clotting or blood pressure. Among the various ways of taking estrogen (pills, patches, vaginal creams, and so on), oral treatment seems to have the best effect on blood lipids. Of course, which form you take may be strongly influenced by other factors, but if lipids are the major concern, oral treatment is the best choice. The patch is second.

There is also some early evidence that certain kinds of progestin have advantages over others, but the research is not yet conclusive enough to make a recommendation.

Q: Does mild hypertension make hormone replacement riskier?
A: Opinion has fluctuated, and there have been times when doctors believed estrogen probably increased blood pressure and thus increased heart disease risk. More recent studies have shown that various hormone replacement methods (cyclic, continuous, estrogen plus progestin) had little or no effect on blood pressure. If you have any questions about your blood pressure,

you absolutely should be evaluated before considering HRT. If your blood pressure is elevated, your doctor will want to monitor it during HRT, but it appears that the reduction of heart disease risk associated with HRT would certainly offset the questionable effect it might have on your blood pressure.

A recent study was described by a former head of the National Institutes of Health as a reason to finally put to rest the "recurrent concern" about HRT's potential cardiovascular side effects. It demonstrated conclusively that HRT did not raise blood pressure, increase the blood's tendency to form clots that could precipitate a stroke or heart attack, or have adverse effects on how the body processes sugar (and thus on the development or exacerbation of diabetes). Some other studies have indicated that estrogen may even have a lowering effect on blood pressure in some women.

Q: Will HRT reactivate my old problem with thrombophlebitis?
A: This is definitely something to be discussed fully with your doctor before starting HRT, particularly if a different doctor treated your phlebitis and your current doctor does not know your history. If it is an "old" problem that has not troubled you recently, HRT is not likely to trigger a recurrence, unless the original problem was associated with pregnancy, use of oral contraceptives, or previous treatment with HRT. If any of those conditions was involved, HRT

should be used with caution and probably with minimum doses of estrogen.

Although there is no conclusive evidence that estrogen increases the danger of clotting, the fact is that age alone increases the risk. Therefore, postmenopausal women are more susceptible to clotting problems than younger women whether they are taking estrogen or not. You should be alert to the signs of a clot and get emergency help immediately if they occur. These signs include sudden or severe headache, sudden loss of co-ordination, sudden loss or change of vision, pains in the chest, groin, or leg (especially in the calf), sudden unexplained shortness of breath, sudden slurring of speech, and weakness or numbness in an arm or leg.

Q: I read somewhere that women who take HRT tend to be healthier and to take better care of their health than women who don't take HRT. Could that account for their lower heart attack rates?

A: This point is often cited in discussions of the value of HRT. There is no clear answer at the moment. What is known is that women with lower blood pressure are more likely to take HRT, as are women in higher economic and educational categories. The latter have a generally lower heart attack risk for reasons not yet identified. It is also obvious that women who take HRT go to their doctors on a more regular basis for monitoring of their treatment and are thus more likely to be tested—and presumably treated—for any risk factors that emerge on these frequent visits. Finally, women who take HRT may be more motivated to take risk-reducing actions than those who do not take HRT. These factors could certainly influence cardiovascular risks independently of any hormone treatment, but if they are not taken into account, the hormones appear to be responsible. On the other hand, HRT's demonstrated beneficial effect on the balance of HDL and LDL in the bloodstream is much more persuasive than the hard-to-prove influence of class and lifestyle. Nevertheless, these unanswered questions underscore the vital importance of thorough assessment, full and open doctor-patient communications, and well-informed decision-making about the relative risks and benefits of HRT for each woman individually.

FOUR

Osteoporosis

CASE STUDY

Catherine, a 58-year-old housewife, had no idea that osteoporosis had weakened her bones until she broke her wrist trying to catch herself during a simple fall. She did not think much about it until I asked about the cast on her arm during her yearly checkup shortly after.

She had begun menopause four years earlier, and since then had experienced only minor discomfort. But she admitted during our talk that she seldom consumed calcium-rich dairy products, had never taken calcium supplements, had smoked until just five years ago, and had been sedentary most of her adult life. All of these things added greatly to her risk of weakened bones later in life.

"I never gave much thought to the possibility of osteoporosis," she told me, "because I've always been pretty healthy. I eat well, and I take vitamins. To me, osteoporosis was something that old ladies got. I know now that I was wrong."

As a result of Catherine's bone-breaking accident, I scheduled her for a dual energy x-ray absorptiometry (DEXA), an extremely accurate procedure that uses very low levels of radiation to measure bone density within the body. The results confirmed my suspicions—Catherine had lost a substantial percentage of total bone mass as a result of menopause and her less than healthful lifestyle. I recommended estrogen-replacement therapy, calcium supplementation, a bone-building medication called alendronate, and regular low-intensity exercise.

If Catherine had been more aware of the risk, she might have discovered that she had a history of osteoporosis in her family. Both her mother and her older sister had been prone to falls and fractures later in life, but no one ever thought that osteoporosis could be the cause. Everyone merely attributed their frequent accidents to "growing older."

Catherine is doing well on ERT and calcium supplementation. A recent DEXA showed a 2 percent increase in body bone mass, and Catherine reports an overall improvement in her health.

Life expectancy for American women has increased by 50 percent in this century, from fifty-one years in 1900 to 79.6 years in 1991. Women are now living much longer after menopause than they used to, and are thus exposed for many more years to the diseases of old age, especially conditions associated with postmenopausal estrogen decline such as osteoporosis. It is a disease that almost exclusively threatens women over age fifty. About half of all postmenopausal women suffer osteoporosis to some degree. The incidence of osteoporosis increases with age, affecting 14.8 percent of women fifty to fifty-nine years of age; 21.6 percent of those aged sixty to sixty-nine; 38.5 percent of those aged seventy to seventy-nine; and 70 percent of women over age eighty.

Many people do not realize that osteoporosis is not only a powerful crippler of women but a killer as well. A woman who has had a severe fracture of the hip because of osteoporosis may be confined to bed. She is thus more vulnerable to blood clots, stroke, pneumonia, and other life-threatening complications. One in every five women who has a hip fracture dies within six months, and 10 to 20 percent die within a year. Osteoporosis kills more women than breast, cervical, and uterine cancer combined.

One problem is that women now approaching or experiencing menopause grew up—and established their health and activity habits—well before the contemporary enthusiasm for fitness, athleticism, good nutrition, and preventive medicine; well before the medical profession reached its current state of knowledge about such crucial matters as the influence of physical activity on the development of osteoporosis. Women now of a menopausal age generally did not play soccer at age ten or go rock climbing in their twenties.

As a result, few of them brought into later life the positive attitudes toward exercise so typical of younger women today. According to a worldwide survey of women reported in the journal *Behavioral Medicine*, women get less exercise than men at all ages and they exercise even less as they get older. A survey of older Americans showed that while many had positive attitudes toward physical activity, most do not put them into action.

Certainly few older American women were told in their teens that they could begin lifelong habits that would help ensure a healthier, happier old age. Unfortunately, they do not appear to be hearing the message even now. One survey showed that seven of ten American women do not know much—if anything—about osteoporosis, and that only a little more than half of women with a graduate or professional education claimed to be very well informed on the subject. This makes women more susceptible to two common myths about osteoporosis. The first is the notion that osteoporosis should not be a concern to anyone under age fifty; the second is that after age fifty it is too late to do anything about it. Both are wrong. Osteoporosis can be prevented if you start in your teens or even twenties, and it can be treated in your forties, fifties, even sixties—if you take the right action before the damage has gone too far.

Q: What is osteoporosis?
A: The term is derived from the Latin for "po-

rous bones." In osteoporosis, the bones become full of holes like a sponge, making them brittle, fragile, not very efficient in supporting weight, and easy to break. Bones are not the hard, solid, unchanging masses most people envision. This may be true of their surfaces, but inside they consist of two very different substances: Half of the bone material is nothing but water; the other half is a mixture of collagen and several minerals, most notably calcium. Bones are constantly growing and changing. From infancy through adolescence, bone is developing; in fact, about 45 percent of all your bone structure is created during your teens. But, throughout life, bone undergoes a process called "remodeling," which means that new bone is being made by the process of creating and storing calcium, while at the same time old bone is removed by the process of breaking down and absorbing calcium. Up until your mid-thirties, the process is in balance: equal amounts are created and destroyed. But after that the breakdown process tends to exceed the buildup, and your bones begin to have less calcium than before. At the same time, your body tends to manufacture less vitamin D, so absorption of calcium to the blood drops off. To maintain normal levels, your bones must release calcium into the bloodstream, thus further lowering the bone calcium. The bones stay the same size, but they become thinner and have larger holes inside them, which makes them lighter and weaker. For most people, the impact of this is simply a little less strength and weight-bearing ability as the years go by.

In osteoporosis, the loss of bone is significant. About 1.3 million older people suffer fractures each year because of it. Millions of others are limited in their activity and mobility, or even incapacitated because the front part of the vertebrae in the spine soften and become compressed, making the spine collapse forward in the familiar "dowager's hump" shape. There is a condition known as "fracture threshold," which means the point at which a bone may be broken by a stress as seemingly trivial as a cough or just picking up a bag of groceries. About half of all women reach this threshold by age sixty-five.

Q: What does estrogen have to do with bones and osteoporosis?

A: Estrogen appears to work in a variety of ways to make bones healthy and keep them that way. At its normal level, it encourages calcium uptake by the bone tissue and blocks the bone-dissolving process. Estrogen preserves bone mineral, apparently by encouraging activity by the osteoblasts—the cells that manufacture new bone. It also appears to block the activity of parathyroid hormone, which tends to dissolve bone. It stimulates the activity of vitamin D, which helps the intestines and kidneys to process calcium. It also stimulates the production and activity of calcitonin, a hormone from the thyroid that protects bones from breakdown. Since estrogen stimulates production of collagen—a binding material—in the skin, it may also do the same in bone, making it stronger and more rigid. Finally, it appears that estrogen stimulates the liver to block the action of certain adrenal hormones that have the ability to dissolve bone.

With age, estrogen begins to decline so that it is not available to counteract the age-related decline in production of new bone. A woman can lose as much as half of her bone substance in the first five years of estrogen deficiency. (Testosterone, which is also involved in the health of bones, does not drop dramatically in the same way, so men are not as susceptible to osteoporosis in their later years as women are.) Estrogen deficiency also means the bonding of elements in the bone structure is weakened.

Q: Does HRT cure osteoporosis?
A: The word "cure" suggests that a treatment corrects an illness permanently. In that sense, the answer is no. But in study after study, estrogen has shown to dramatically slow down or stop the rate of bone loss and to drastically cut the occurrence of hip fractures an average of 50 percent. Certain specialists have reported a 90 percent reduction in compression fractures of the spine resulting in dowager's hump among women who took estrogen for ten years.

Q: What are the symptoms of osteoporosis?
A: Unfortunately, there are not any apparent symptoms until the damage is done. A woman or a member of her family may notice that she

seems a little shorter. More often, osteoporosis is discovered only when a bone breaks. It is relatively easy to determine whether a person who has a fracture in later life has osteoporosis because the X ray looks different from that of an ordinary fracture.

Q: Why do older people seem to fall so much?
A: They do not "seem" to fall so much; they really do. About one-third of all people over sixty-five fall some time during the course of a year, frequently in the winter. Surprisingly, it is not because of snow and ice; winter falls, like those occuring in other seasons, happen mostly indoors. It is not definite, but the theory is that in the winter there is less sunlight, which may lead to some kind of neuromuscular deficit, perhaps akin to seasonal affective disorder or "winter blues." People are perhaps just less steady on their feet as a result. Other contributing factors are poor eyesight, poor balance because of hearing loss, muscle weakness due to lack of exercise, and various illnesses of old age.

Q: How often do falls cause fractures?
A: About 1 percent of all falls among people over sixty-five involve a fracture. What most people do not realize is that osteoporosis is itself a cause of falls; when calcium loss is severe and the bones are filled with more air than solid material, a weight-bearing bone such as the femoral head (hip) can break spontaneously—that is, from the slightest stress, and the person loses balance and

falls. In such cases, the fracture causes the accident, not the other way round.

Q: What are the most common fractures?
A: Definitely the hip, by a wide margin. Of all hip fractures in the United States, 90 percent are among people over age fifty. Of those, 80 percent are among women. Wrist fractures become increasingly common as women go from age forty to sixty-five, then the rate levels off. In men, the rate is constant from age twenty to eighty.

It is ironic that one of several reasons why these particular bones—or rather joints—are so susceptible to fracture is that they were so well designed for their normal function. There are actually two major kinds of bone in the body. The outer part of bones is compact bone, which is solid and hard. The inside is spongy bone called cancellous or trabecular bone—meaning that they have a latticelike structure. The spine, wrist, and hip have a larger proportion of the latter than all the other bones. This makes them excellent shock absorbers; if they were solid throughout, every step, every movement, would jar the body from heel to head. Leaning on your elbow would send a shock to your shoulder, and doing a handstand would be terribly painful. At the same time, this makes such bones more vulnerable to the effects of estrogen depletion. The holes between the latticework get bigger, the connections between fibers in the lattice get broken, and the bones become fragile—they no longer absorb shock, but are broken by it.

Q: What are the most important risk factors for osteoporosis?

A: The two most obvious are getting older and being a woman. (By age sixty-five, the average man still has 90 percent of his peak bone mass, a woman only 74 percent.) Poor eating habits, especially a calcium-poor diet, are of major importance. Other risk factors—not in order of significance—include being chronically underweight, having a family history of osteoporosis, sedentary habits, smoking, and heavy drinking. Long-term overreplacement with thyroid hormone is a risk factor. Women who are taking cortisone for asthma, rheumatoid arthritis, or other conditions are susceptible because these medications tend to weaken the spongy bone.

An interesting aspect of risk is that Caucasian women are considerably more susceptible than women of African ancestry. There is no accepted scientific explanation for this; one suggested theory is that a genetic advantage resulted from living in an area of strong year-round sunshine, which stimulates production of Vitamin D—an important bone-builder. Races evolving in the northern hemisphere were deprived of adequate ultraviolet light much of the year.

Q: Being chronically underweight is a risk factor for osteoporosis, but aren't chronically overweight people also more at risk if they try to lose weight late in life?

A: There is some evidence from one scientific study suggesting that any woman who loses an appreciable amount of weight after age fifty increases her risk. But the woman who has always been lean increases hers more. In this study of more than 3,600 women over age 67, current weight was compared with what the women said they weighed when they were age fifty, then rates of osteoporosis were calculated. The women were described in three weight categories: lean (5 foot 4, and weighing 110 pounds at age fifty), average (5 foot 4, 140 pounds), and heavyset (5 foot 4 and 175 pounds). A lean woman who lost 5 percent of her body weight increased her risk twofold over a lean woman whose weight remained the same. An average-weight or heavyset woman increased her risk twofold if she lost 10 percent of her body weight. The leaner woman is still at a greater disadvantage. One reason is that naturally lean women simply have less bone mass to begin with, so any loss of bone will have a greater impact. Another is that lean women produce less estrogen. To make matters worse, lean women are more susceptible to fractures if they do have osteoporosis, because they have less body fat to cushion their bones from falls or trauma.

Another interesting aspect of this study was that the scientists did not ask the women why they decided to lose weight at that particular time in their lives, or whether they lost weight by reducing food intake or increasing exercise. The scientists said it did not matter which way the weight was lost: exercise helps build bones but weight loss from any cause always means bone loss, and apparently the weight loss has a greater negative impact than the positive effect of the exercise.

Q: Can I do anything to cut the risk?
A: Absolutely, if you take action before osteoporosis becomes established. Prevention consists of beginning in adolescence to insure sufficient intake of calcium along with a lifetime commitment to exercise. Whether you have done that or not, around the time of menopause you can do several things to stave off the process.

First, get sufficient calcium in your diet. The general daily recommended allowance is 800 mg. Adolescent and young adult women, pregnant women, or nursing mothers should get 1,200 mg daily. After menopause, 1,500 is recommended and 1,750 considered even more ideal. Most American women are calcium deficient, averaging about half a gram a day. At menopause, a woman loses about a gram and a half a day, leaving the average woman a whole gram short. It is important to remember that even adequate calcium intake will not deter osteoporosis if you are noticeably estrogen-deficient.

Second, exercise regularly. It is been demonstrated that certain kinds of physical activity not only slows down bone loss but actually encourages bone building. The best exercises are those that put some stress or pressure on bones, which strengthens them the same way exercise strengthens muscle. Walking, climbing stairs, aerobic exercise or dance, racket sports, and bi-

cycling are all good exercises that can be done at
appropriate levels at almost any age. But strenuous, prolonged stress such as long-distance run-
ning can cause more harm than good to the
bones.

Third, eliminate bad health habits that are detrimental to bones: smoking, alcohol, excessive
caffeine, and certain prescription and over-the-
counter medications, which you should discuss
with your doctor. Cigarette smoking not only increases the loss of bone and raises the likelihood
of osteoporosis, but it appears to hasten menopause; women who smoke go through menopause an average of two or three years earlier
than those who do not. Too much alcohol (that
is, more than one or two drinks a day regularly)
also reduces bone mass; it also interferes with the
building of bone and the processing of vitamin
D, which builds bone. Excessive drinking is usually associated with poor nutrition, which is also
detrimental to bone health. Caffeine interferes
with healthy processing of calcium.

Fourth, watch your general nutrition, especially vitamin D, and especially in the winter if
you live in the northern hemisphere. Sunshine is
the natural stimulant to vitamin D production,
but it is difficult to get enough sun in the winter—and sunscreens in summer will impede vitamin D production. Foods containing vitamin D
include butter, eggs, liver, fatty fish, and fortified
milk—often foods that are avoided in today's fat-
conscious diet. Vitamin supplements can bring
you up to the recommended 400 IU (Interna-

tional Units) per day, but too much more than that can have a negative effect.

Q: If I'm already approaching menopause, can I still prevent osteoporosis?
A: Yes—even if you are menopausal or postmenopausal, so long as osteoporosis is not already established.

Q: Where should I get calcium?
A: Some examples of good sources and the amounts they provide include low-fat milk, 298 mg per cup (eight ounces); skim milk, 303 mg per cup; yogurt, 300 to 450 mg a cup; broccoli and kale are also good sources. Skim milk and low-fat yogurt are recommended because they contain little fat, and also contain vitamin D and lactose, which help the body utilize the calcium. Other good sources are herring, salmon, sardines (if you eat the little bones), and tofu. Hard cheeses, such as Swiss or American, contain calcium but also have a lot of salt, cholesterol, and saturated fat. Cottage cheese has less of those but very little calcium. Other calcium sources, containing 100 to 150 calories per serving, include chili with beans, scallops, shrimp, spinach, turnip greens, dried figs, pizza, and seedless raisins.

Q: Do calcium supplements or antacid tablets containing calcium help prevent osteoporosis?
A: For some time, scientists could not demonstrate that calcium supplements had the same effect as calcium obtained from food. In the past

three or four years, solid scientific evidence has demonstrated that supplements do help even in postmenopausal women. One study suggested that supplements significantly increased bone density in women who also got regular exercise. In 1993, the *Archives of Internal Medicine*, a medical journal, reported that calcium supplements retard bone loss and should be considered a useful strategy in helping prevent early postmenopausal osteoporosis. Of course, it is almost universally agreed that the best way to get calcium is through your diet. But supplements are a sure way of getting enough calcium for those whose eating habits are not consistent or who do not always remember they are supposed to eat certain calcium-containing foods every day. The goal is to get at least 750 mg from food. A woman could get this much from a glass of skim milk, one serving of kale or other dark leafy green vegetable, and a serving of low-fat yogurt a day. If she takes a 1,000 mg calcium supplement her total will be a healthy 1,750 mg. Certain antacid tablets do contain calcium but you might have to take more than the recommended daily limit in order to meet calcium needs, unless you are getting a lot of calcium in your food. This is something to check with your doctor.

Q: If there are no warning symptoms, how do I find out if I need to be doing something about osteoporosis?

A: If you are approaching or undergoing menopause, you should already be doing something about it: getting appropriate exercise and making sure your calcium intake is sufficient. But, to discover whether you might need some other form of treatment, such as HRT, you can ask your doctor about a special kind of x-ray examination called bone densitometry—or dual energy x-ray absorptiometry (DEXA). This reveals the most significant sign of osteoporosis: whether your bone mass is significantly below peak level— peak level being that which is found in a woman in her early twenties. The amount of reduction in bone mass density (BMD) is measured by what scientists call "standard deviation," and for each of these units below peak, the risk of fracture increases two to two-and-a-half times. But if a woman has already had a fracture, her risk of another fracture is twenty-five times that of another woman who has the same degree of bone mass loss but who has not had a fracture yet. Unfortunately, by the time a woman starts fracturing bones, it is too late to make a really major impact on the disease by any form of treatment. The best measures are early diagnosis and prevention. If you are of menopausal age, and especially if you are having any menopausal symptoms, you should be seeing your physician for a general physical checkup that includes bone densitometry if possible. The DEXA procedure takes between fifteen and forty-five minutes and uses such a low level of x-ray power that the technician remains in the room instead of retreating behind a lead shield as in other x-ray examinations. It costs between $150 and $300,

depending on your location. Insurance coverage—
or lack of it—varies widely depending on the insurance company and geography. It might not be
available in your area since there are only about
1,500 DEXA machines in the U.S., but there are
some alternative procedures; these measure bone
density but not as precisely as DEXA.

**Q: How long do I have to take estrogen supple-
ments to protect myself against osteoporosis?**
A: There is some debate about this because different research has produced different data. The
well-known Framingham study showed that
women under age seventy-five who had taken
long-term estrogen therapy had higher bone density than those who had not, but after age
seventy-five there was little difference. There is
considerably more controversy over the question
of bone density after stopping HRT. Some research shows that it drops rapidly; others that it
does not. What is definitely known is that without HRT, bone density decreases by 2 percent a
year for the first five years after menopause, then
by 1 percent a year. This means that bone density
decreases by 30 percent from age fifty to eighty.
It has been suggested that the options for women
are to take HRT indefinitely to guarantee that
there will be no further decrease after stopping
therapy; to take it only after osteoporosis has
been clearly demonstrated, by a fracture, for instance; or to take it for ten years, which is often
not acceptable to women. Like so many other aspects of women's health, especially menopause

and estrogen, this should be a highly individual decision, based on your doctor's knowledge of your health, tests such as bone density, your symptoms, your lifestyle and preferences, and most of all the extent of your understanding of the overall impact of various options.

Q: Is estrogen the only medical treatment for osteoporosis?
A: No. There are several nonhormonal drugs that have been used as alternatives (or sometimes supplements) to hormone treatment. Calcium slows bone loss to some extent and appears to reduce the incidence of fractures. Calcium plus vitamin D also increases density of some bones and lowers fracture rates, while vitamin D alone seems to protect bone but not reduce fractures. Some studies have suggested that calcitonin, a human thyroid hormone, may do the same thing, although the statistics regarding its ability to prevent fractures are inconclusive. A number of studies do support the suggestion that calcitonin helps relieve pain in osteoporotic fractures of the vertebrae. It is relatively expensive.

There are two nonhormonal compounds that are now in the early stage of being used for osteoporosis. One is called etidronate, one of the class of drugs called biphosphonates, which chemically resemble a natural substance in the body that is involved in the storage and removal of calcium in bone. The compound is usually given in cycles alternately with calcium supplements over a ninety-day period; the dose is one etidronate tablet a day for fourteen days, then a 500 mg calcium tablet every day for seventy-six days. This cycle is then repeated. It appears to help stave off osteoporosis by preventing the osteoclasts (or bone-removers) from absorbing and breaking down bone. Studies have shown that etidronate does increase the spinal bone density of early-menopausal and postmenopausal women who have not yet developed osteoporosis, and after two years of treatment, the rate of expected fractures had been cut in half.

Etidronate has been approved by the FDA only for the treatment of Paget's disease (which is similar to osteoporosis in that it involves the breakdown of bone) and for prevention of abnormal bone development after hip replacement and spinal cord injury. It has already been approved for use in osteoporosis in Canada, Australia, and a number of European countries. It is still classified as a research drug in the U.S., where its generally accepted use as a treatment for osteoporosis has declined with the emergence of alendronate, another member of the biphosphonate class.

Alendronate has recently been studied in women with reduced bone mass. It appears to be about a thousand times more potent than etidronate in inhibiting the breakdown of bone. This means it can be taken in lower doses, which might offset any dangers of accumulation. In the first major study of this new drug, more than nine hundred postmenopausal women took a daily dose of alendronate plus 500 mg of calcium daily for five years, at which point they averaged more than an 8 percent increase in spinal bone mass with somewhat smaller increases in other bones. Their fracture rate was half that of a group of women who took a placebo or dummy pill.

What makes these medications most interesting is that they not only prevent further bone loss in women who already have osteoporosis but also seem to restore lost bone mass—something that has always been much harder to do. The major drawback is that biphosphonates tend to accumulate in the bone, and it is not yet known what long-term effect this may have. It might prevent the healing of microscopic fractures which are fairly common among the elderly.

Q: **If I choose to try HRT for bone loss prevention, when's the best time to start?**
A: It is most beneficial if begun during or right after menopause. HRT seems to have little or no effect after age seventy-five—which of course is the time of highest risk. As with prevention, it is a case of "the sooner the better."

Q: **Is there a difference—in dosage, for example—between hormone replacement for osteoporosis and HRT for menopausal symptoms like hot flashes?**
A: Not really, except for individual differences in symptoms, needs, metabolism, and many other factors. For example, if you are beginning estro-

gen treatment at the time of menopause, the "standard" dose of one particular brand is 0.625 to 1.25 mg, although some women are not relieved of hot flashes at the lowest end of that dosage scale. The word "standard" is quoted to emphasize again the importance of individually tailored treatment. Two women on the same dose may have entirely different results: one may not be relieved of her symptoms at all because she burns up estrogen at a much higher rate; the other may have symptoms of excessive dosage, such as bloating, weight gain, and early or heavy bleeding because she does not process the estrogen as efficiently. For most women, the lower dosage (0.625 milligrams) is enough to protect the bones from calcium loss—but any less than that is inadequate, and some women may need more.

Q: **What's the difference between osteoporosis and osteoarthritis, and is the latter also a problem after menopause?**
A: Osteoarthritis is a chronic inflammation of the joints. Unlike osteoporosis, in which bone is destroyed and which is painless, osteoarthritis is painful and occurs when cartilage is broken down, bone overgrows areas where it should not, and bony spurs may form. What it has in common with osteoporosis is that postmenopausal women are most at risk for developing this disease and that estrogen appears to play an important role. It is also a major contributor to hip fractures; it accounts for more than 70 percent of

the 200,000 hip and knee replacement operations performed each year in the United States.

Early results from clinical trials suggest that estrogen appears to protect against osteoarthritis as it does against osteoporosis. A recent study of 4,366 white women age sixty-five and older (black women were excluded because they rarely fracture their hips) showed that women who were currently taking HRT had a lower rate of osteoarthritis (less than nine percent) than those who had never taken it (13 percent). The reduction was found only in women who were still taking estrogen or who had taken it for at least ten years before this study. Women who had been taking estrogen for one to ten years had a rate of about 10 percent. Women who had once taken estrogen but had quit before ten years time had the same rate of osteoarthritis as women who had never taken hormones (13 percent).

FIVE

❦

Drug Therapy

CASE STUDY

Noreen, a 56-year-old nurse in a hospital intensive care unit, came to me seeking HRT to alleviate the medium to severe symptoms she was experiencing from menopause, particularly mood swings and frequent hot flashes. As a health care professional, Noreen was knowledgeable about HRT and felt she was a good candidate for its use. She was fairly certain her symptoms were the result of estrogen deficiency.

I examined Noreen and quickly confirmed what she had told me. She was about two years into menopause, and lab tests showed a marked decrease in her estrogen levels. I prescribed a standard dose, long-acting estrogen supplement and asked her for a follow-up call in one month.

But a week after Noreen started the patch, she called me complaining of nausea, persistent headaches, insomnia, and a mild, itchy skin rash. "I have a pretty good threshold for problems like these," she told me, "but I don't think I can take much more. These side effects are worse than the symptoms of my menopause."

I scheduled Noreen for a follow-up visit the next day, suspecting that the specific type and high dosage of estrogen she was receiving was the cause of her complaints. A blood test confirmed this; Noreen was one of a small percentage of patients who are extremely sensitive to hormone therapy. With a better understanding of her needs, I switched her to a different type of estrogen in a lower dosage.

A follow-up visit two weeks later revealed a much happier patient. The side effects had disappeared within days, and the new therapy was slowly but surely reducing the severity of Noreen's menopause symptoms.

"I was more than a little concerned," Noreen said later. "I really wanted this therapy to work, and I was afraid that the side effects would prevent me from using HRT."

Estrogen and other hormones play a key role in a woman's health throughout life. During menopause there is a loss of hormones that results in a wide range of symptoms that vary in duration and intensity—from dry skin to depression. Women are also susceptible in later life to certain diseases such as osteoporosis and heart disease due in part to the absence of estrogen's protective effects. After weighing the risks and benefits for themselves under the supervision and guidance of a skilled physician, some women choose to manage their menopause by using HRT, which is normally a combination of estrogen and the hormone progestin. Other women decide that their medical history and other factors make the use of these therapies too risky, or they think that the dwindling down of their reproductive capability is inevitable and somehow a part of nature's "scheme of things"—and should not be artificially manipulated. That does not mean that they are doomed to suffer for the span of a decade at the whims of their bodies' unpredictable march towards maturity. It simply means that they must examine other treatment options, including alternative treatments, and lifestyle changes if they want some measure of relief from their symptoms and protection against serious illnesses.

To learn about HRT, it is important to make a distinction between hormone therapy that adds hormones and therapy that replaces them. The first form of therapy, which adds hormones even if yours are not inadequate, consists of contraceptive pills, which may be used for purposes other than birth control. For example, they can smooth out irregularities in menstrual periods or occasionally relieve premenstrual syndrome. The second form, HRT, is designed to put back some of the hormones you may be missing to counteract the ill effects of estrogen deficiency. HRT is given to women who have hormone imbalances from various causes, but it's primarily used by women during menopause.

Q: What hormones are in oral contraceptives?
A: Almost all contain essentially the same two ingredients. The most significant is estrogen, the hormone you naturally secrete throughout your entire menstrual cycle. Two different estrogens may be used: ethinyl estradiol and mestranol. These are versions of the estrogens your body produces normally that have been chemically modified so that they are effective when taken by mouth (unlike natural estrogen). The other ingredient is progestin, a form of progesterone, which your body produces in large amounts only during the second half of the menstrual cycle to prepare the lining of the uterus for implantation and pregnancy.

Q: How do birth control pills work?
A: As we have seen in discussing how estrogen works throughout your life, there is a complicated feedback or communications loop involving your pituitary gland and various hormones, including estrogen, progesterone, and (most crucially for contraception) FSH. Oral contraceptives provide enough additional estrogen and progesterone to "trick" the pituitary gland so that it does not produce the surge of FSH that usually occurs midway in your menstrual cycle. Without FSH, the ovarian follicles do not release eggs, and without eggs, there can be no pregnancy. Oral contraceptives also regulate menstrual bleeding.

Q: **How do doctors decide on the dosage?**
A: The basic idea is to give the smallest amount of estrogen that will be effective; no more, no less. For obvious practical reasons, oral contraceptives are designed for the "average" woman; that is, the amount of estrogen they contain is based on the amount of estrogen the average healthy woman produces naturally at mid-menstrual cycle. Since not every woman is average, some women require an adjustment of the dosage or even the balance of hormones in the pill. But for most women the standard dosage does the job intended without creating any problems.

Q: **What does "low-dose pill" mean?**
A: The first birth control pills contained as much as 100 micrograms of estrogen, in the belief that this much was needed to prevent the FSH surge. But after years of experience it was learned that it does not require much estrogen to suppress FSH—just more than the woman's normal estrogen level. Today's contraceptive pills contain only 20 to 35 micrograms of estrogen. What many people still do not understand is that most of the problems with the early contraceptives (such as breakthrough bleeding or other menstrual abnormalities) were due to the high dosage of estrogen, not to the basic action of contraceptive pills.

Q: **Is there any difference between brands of oral contraceptives?**

A: Definitely. The major differences are in the pill-taking schedule followed and the type of progestin used. There are at least half a dozen different versions of progestin now used in oral contraceptives, some differing only very slightly. The most noticeable difference is that some are less androgenic than others; that is, they have fewer "masculinizing" effects (such as skin or hair problems). The so-called newer progestins are quite different from the old standards. These forms of progestin (norgestimate and desogestrel) are considerably less androgenic. In addition, they do not have an unfavorable effect on your lipid levels (a problem with some older progestins) and seem to cause fewer problems with excessive or off-schedule bleeding. This does not mean that if you are taking one of the traditional oral contraceptives, you should rush to your doctor and ask for the "newer" model. If the one you are using works without causing you problems, stick with it.

Q: Why are oral contraceptives used for acne, unwanted facial hair, and female baldness?

A: The emphasis in this book is on hormone replacement for menopause and other symptoms of estrogen deficiency. But there is an associated hormonal imbalance that causes problems for many women; that is, an excess of androgens (so-called "male" hormones) relative to estrogens ("female" hormones). Because oral contraceptives are designed to smooth out and "normalize" the balance of hormones, they can often relieve symptoms of androgen excess such as the ones above.

Q: Are oral contraceptives useful for women who don't have regular periods?

A: Yes, depending on the reason for irregularity. Missed periods can have many causes, including malnutrition, emotional problems, excessive exercise, various systemic diseases, and, of course, estrogen deficiency—which also has a variety of causes. Irregular periods should be evaluated, not dismissed lightly. Oral contraceptives or HRT (estrogen and progestin replacement) can correct some of the causes of irregularity.

Q: Do birth control pills or hormone replacement relieve PMS?

A: This is controversial. Experts almost universally agree that hormones cause premenstrual syndrome (PMS). But they almost universally disagree about whether hormone treatment—at least the treatment now available—really works. The problem, as often noted in this book, is that women's hormonal health is extremely individual and sometimes complicated. It is often hard to know exactly what hormonal problem may be causing any particular woman's PMS. And of course there are various neurotransmitters—nerve signal messengers—and brain chemicals that are involved with mood and emotion. Some women are just more susceptible to low moods because of their natures, and life situations can exaggerate PMS at times. At the moment, there are not specific tests that can tell us exactly what is going on chemically when you have PMS. And without knowing what is out of balance, it is difficult to fashion a specific treatment. What you—and your doctor—can do is to experiment. Your knowledge about your symptoms and moods, combined with your doctor's expertise and experience with other patients, can be put together into any one of several different approaches that are worth trying. Basically, a good approach is to start with the simplest treatment and move on to those more complex if the first does not work. For example, some women are helped by simple changes in diet and lifestyle (see Chapter 8, "The Alternatives"). Counseling, exercise, retraining yourself to have better sleeping habits, and avoiding or relieving stress may not remove the symptoms but could make them far more tolerable. Biofeedback training or relaxation training have helped some women. Those with a tendency toward low mood may be helped by antidepressant medication if there is no obstacle to taking it. (For example, if there is an indication of potential alcohol or prescription drug abuse, antidepressants should be considered with great caution.)

Q: How is HRT different from contraceptive hormone therapy?
A: Essentially, oral contraceptives are designed to raise the levels of estrogen and progestin *above* normal; that is, they *add* hormones to those that are already there. HRT is designed to counteract

a reduced level of estrogen; it replaces *missing* hormones. The rate at which estrogen levels drop during menopause may greatly influence how comfortable or uncomfortable a woman may be, the severity of her symptoms, or whether she has any problems at all. There is a major difference in the dosage of estrogen used for contraception and the amount used for menopausal symptoms. As previously discussed, today's birth control pills contain about 30 to 35 micrograms of estrogen, a relatively small amount compared to early doses of 80 to 100 micrograms. Postmenopausal women are considered estrogen deficient when their blood level of estrogen drops below 60 micrograms. (A man's level is 70.) This level of estrogen (60 micrograms) is needed to prevent osteoporosis; 100 micrograms are needed to protect your cardiovascular system. Typical "replacement" dosages of estrogen may range from 60 to 150 micrograms, depending on many factors. The higher doses may be used for severe menopausal symptoms such as night sweats, insomnia, and irritability.

Q: I've almost stopped having menstrual periods although I have no other menopausal symptoms. Should I have my estrogen level checked?

A: Not unless your gynecologist or primary care physician sees some other reason to do so. The important thing about estrogen levels appears to be not just how high or low they are before and during menopause, but how dramatically the estrogen level drops at menopause. Thus, a woman who has relatively low levels of estrogen before menopause and whose levels do not drop very far at menopause may not have symptoms as pronounced as a woman who has high levels that drop markedly. As discussed elsewhere, there are also other influences on menstrual symptoms that are completely unrelated to estrogen level.

Q: What hormones are used in HRT?
A: Estrogen, of course, is the main component. In fact, for many years it was the only ingredient. Today, estrogen replacement therapy (ERT) is almost never used alone except in women who have had a hysterectomy. The other significant ingredient in HRT is progestin, which was added because it has been found to protect against endometrial hyperplasia (abnormalities in the uterine lining). Before menopause, estrogen stimulates the enrichment of the lining of the uterus in preparation for receiving a fertilized egg. If no egg is implanted, progestin then steps in and makes the uterine lining (endometrium) shed its extra cells, which produces menstrual bleeding. If menopausal women took only estrogen, the endometrium would continue to build up, which results in endometrial abnormalities and greatly increases the risk of endometrial cancer. This was the great drawback of earlier estrogen-only treatments. Progestin is also very effective against hot flashes and may help preserve bone density.

Q: Is progestin ever used alone?
A: In early menopause when your periods begin to become irregular or abnormal, both ovulation and progesterone production are slowing down. At this time, progestin is sometimes given to help control the irregularity and prevent uterine hyperplasia. But estrogen levels may still be high so there would be no point in replacing estrogen. Progestin alone may also be used for women whose chief symptom is hot flashes, who also want to preserve bone density, and for whom estrogen is contraindicated.

Q: If I try hormone replacement and decide to stop, will that cause any harm?
A: First, it is absolutely essential that you do not stop suddenly. Normally, at menopause, most women's estrogen levels decline over a period of time (in some women, this decline may happen more quickly than in others, but never abruptly except for surgical menopause). If your natural levels have gone way down but are being kept high by hormone replacement, stopping treatment would mean an instant drop in estrogen, which could cause symptoms much worse than the ones you were trying to treat. Your hot flashes would probably become quite severe. But carefully supervised cessation of hormone replacement will not damage your health in other ways. The important point here is, what is your reason for taking hormone replacement to begin with? If you are simply concerned with hot flashes and other menopausal symptoms, you

may want to take hormones only for the acute menopausal period and taper off at the time you would naturally be coming out of menopause. If you want the long-term protection HRT provides against heart disease, osteoporosis, and other consequences of low estrogen, then you should continue with the treatment.

Q: What kind of protection does long-term HRT provide?

A: It is estimated that if you take HRT for ten years from the beginning of menopause you reduce your risk of osteoporotic fracture and heart attack by half, and your risk of stroke may be cut by about a third.

Q: I've heard that HRT is good for your teeth. Is that true?

A: One study of 42,000 postmenopausal women showed that those who have used female hormones regularly at some time were one-fourth as likely to lose their teeth than those who never used HRT.

Q: What are "unopposed estrogens?"

A: This simply means estrogens given alone, without any progestin to "oppose" some of the effects of estrogen (for example, accumulation of abnormal uterine lining). Today, because of what is now understood about the risks of unopposed estrogen, estrogen-only treatment is reserved almost exclusively for women who no longer have a uterus and therefore do not need the progestin that is added to HRT in order to prevent diseases of the uterus.

Q: How often do I have to take hormones?
A: That depends on the method your doctor recommends. Some of the information you may have read about HRT may make it sound as if treatment can be very complicated—and, in fact, it can be. But there are really only a few very basic methods, and most schedules follow one of them. They include unopposed estrogen, cyclic combined therapy, and continuous combined therapy.

Unopposed estrogen, as explained previously, is estrogen not modified or diluted by the progestin that is used in most forms of HRT. A woman who has undergone a hysterectomy (removal of the uterus) obviously is in no danger of uterine cancer and does not need the protection expected from the added progestin.

Cyclic combined therapy administers estrogen and progestin over an appropriate number of days to simulate the hormonal fluctuations of a natural menstrual cycle. Actually, there are two variations on this theme. In one method, estrogen is given throughout the entire month with progestin added only for the first twelve days of the cycle. On the twelfth day, bleeding occurs; this is considered a normal cycle. Bleeding at any other time requires medical evaluation for endometrial abnormalities. In the second method, estrogen is given for the first twenty-five days of the month and progestin is given from the fourteenth to the twenty-fifth day. For one week—the last week of the month, after progestin is given—no hormone is taken. Bleeding should begin on the twenty-fifth day; if it occurs earlier than this, endometrial testing is required. Physicians base their use of this approach on long-standing concerns about giving estrogen continuously to menopausal women, but most of these concerns are based on outdated approaches. Others cite more recent evidence that there is no harm in continuous dosing of estrogen and that dropping estrogen for a week can cause the sudden return of hot flashes. These are decisions that should be made individually by a woman and her doctor.

Continuous combined therapy is a common choice. The standard practice is to give low doses of the most commonly prescribed form of estrogen (conjugated equine estrogen) and progestin (medroprogesterone acetate) every day. Various other combinations of estrogen and progestin may be used. Although there are no large statistical studies showing whether this method has great advantages or disadvantages compared to cyclic therapy, studies that have been performed do indicate one major difference: A considerably greater majority of women taking continuous therapy compared with those on cyclic therapy stop having any menstrual bleeding at all. One study showed that about 80 percent to 90 percent of women taking cyclic hormones still have periods, compared with only 25 percent of women taking continuous treatment.

Q: Are there different ways of taking HRT?
A: There are many different ways. First of all, there are various schedules for taking oral hormone replacement. Then there are many different dosage forms of hormones, including patches, creams, gels, and injections. Each form has its particular advantages and disadvantages, and treatment should be tailored to each individual woman depending on her needs, problems, risks, and comfort.

Q: What's the advantage of pills?
A: Most of all, they are convenient. And they can be given on various different schedules that meet each individual's needs. Their disadvantage is that they tend to increase estrogen levels right after you take them and decrease levels as it gets closer to the time for the next dose. The ideal is to have a reliable steady level of estrogen over time. This is not a major problem for most people. About one woman in twenty has some digestive or metabolic characteristic that keeps oral estrogen from properly entering her system, so although she is taking pills, she tests low for estrogen, regardless of her dosage. In this instance, one of the various other forms can be tried.

Q: I have a history of gallbladder disease that my doctor says would interfere with my using hormone pills. Why is that?
A: Oral estrogen can cause an unwanted increase in certain lipids if you have gallbladder prob-

lems. Other forms of hormone administration such as a patch do not cause this difficulty.

Q: What's good about the hormone patch?
A: The patch is also called "transdermal therapeutic system" or TTP, because it releases hormones transdermally (through the skin). The patch is paper-thin, about the size of a half-dollar, and quite simple to use. You put it on your back, buttocks, or stomach. With certain brands, you remove the old patch twice a week and put a new one on a different spot. Some of the newer brands are changed only once a week. Patches are generally convenient and have the advantage of releasing hormones evenly over a period of time, instead of releasing high levels that taper off, as pills do. A few women are bothered by skin rashes from patch use. Although the patches should not fall off even when wet, some women do lose them when bathing, showering, exercising, swimming, or sweating. You can put the same patch right back on or put on a new one.

Q: How do estrogen creams work?
A: Estrogen creams are inserted into the vagina at bedtime with an applicator, like a spermicidal contraceptive foam. While the estrogen is absorbed into your circulation through the vaginal walls, it softens and lubricates the walls, which is an advantage for women who are bothered by severe vaginal dryness. Estrogen creams work in the same way as oral hormones or transdermal

patches, but they are effective in much lower doses than these other forms, making them a good choice for women who do not want or cannot take high levels of estrogen. For example, even women with a history or risk of breast cancer can use this form of hormone replacement. But the procedure is somewhat untidy, the cream can leak out during the night, and some women find the applicator unpleasant or inconvenient.

Q: What are the advantages of tablets and rings?
A: Vaginal tablets are placed internally like a cream about three times a week. Their major benefit is that this form of hormone is sometimes absorbed so efficiently that the dose can be kept to an extremely low level and still be effective in combating symptoms. Vaginal rings are inserted like a diaphragm and left in place for three months at a time. They are not currently available in the United States.

Q: What's the difference between creams and gels?
A: The creams are mostly vaginal. Skin gels, which are applied to the upper body every day, are largely a European product not yet available in the United States.

Q: Which women get the most benefit from implants?
A: Implants are rarely used except in women who have had their ovaries removed. They consist of pellets of pure crystals of estrogen, each about the size of a grain of wheat. In a relatively

simple office procedure, they are placed under the skin of the abdominal wall, near the groin. The pellets are made to release estrogen slowly and evenly into the bloodstream over a number of months. This has the advantage of convenience and of providing an even supply of estrogen, but there can be problems. Fibrous or stringy tissue developing at the implant site can slow absorption and require replacement of the implants at another site. Women with implants have to be careful about overheating at the implant site—for example, through using a heating pad or hot water bottle—because this can speed up absorption and make the estrogen level too high.

Q: What's the difference between ovariectomy and total hysterectomy or partial hysterectomy?
A: The differences are extremely important for many reasons, but particularly in regard to HRT. There are several different kinds of surgery involving the reproductive system, and only the three that entail removal of both ovaries (with or without fallopian tubes, and with or without removal of the uterus) create what is called "surgical menopause," caused by the abrupt and total cessation of estrogen production. This requires hormone replacement. The kinds of surgery are as follows.

- *Ovariectomy or oophorectomy* is the removal of a single ovary. The other remains in place and functioning, so that if you are premenopausal, you still produce hormones, still ovulate, can become pregnant, and will experience natural menopause.

- *Simple hysterectomy* is the removal of the uterus and sometimes the fallopian tubes, which are attached to it. Ovaries are not affected, so if you are premenopausal, you are still producing hormones. Women who have simple hysterectomies do stop having menstrual periods, which often deceives them into thinking that they have undergone menopause.

- *Total hysterectomy* is the removal of the uterus and the cervix. The ovaries are still in place, hormones are produced, and no surgical menopause occurs. This is a term that causes a great deal of confusion, because it has become widely—and wrongly—understood among women to mean removal of *all* the essential reproductive organs: uterus, cervix, both ovaries, and the fallopian tubes.

- *Hysterectomy with bilateral salpingo-oophorectomy* is the correct medical terminology for the removal of the uterus, cervix, both ovaries, and the fallopian tubes. It causes instant surgical menopause.

- *Bilateral oophorectomy* is removal of both ovaries but not the fallopian tubes. It is the second kind of surgery that creates surgical menopause.

- *Bilateral salpingo-oophorectomy* is removal of both ovaries and fallopian tubes. This is the third form of surgical menopause.

Q: I had a simple hysterectomy in my late thirties. Now that I'm approaching menopause, what can I expect?

A: Your ovaries, presumably, have been producing estrogen all along even if you have not been menstruating, but the levels have probably been declining. Eventually you should have a natural menopause, although you may not even be aware of it if you do not have hot flashes or other symptoms, because you will not go through the irregular menstruation and eventual cessation of menstruation that other menopausal women do. You will, of course, be subject to the same postmenopausal risks as other women, and may wish to consider hormone replacement on the same basis—for protection, not symptom relief.

Q: Does surgical menopause carry any special risks?

A: That depends on whether you are talking about symptoms or long-term health dangers such as heart disease. Certainly, the instant loss of all estrogen causes a dramatic health change. The sudden menopausal symptoms, if not treated, can be more severe than those that arrive slowly over time. The other issue is that menopause due to surgery usually occurs earlier than natural menopause would have, so that you face the increased health risks earlier and for a longer period of time. Women who have had their ovaries removed before natural menopause are estimated to face seven times the risk of heart disease of those who go through menopause naturally. The risk of osteoporosis also speeds up. You can offset some of these dangers with diet, exercise, and other alternative measures, but most doctors agree that women who have had surgical menopause have a special need for the protective effects of HRT.

Q: Is there any difference between synthetic and natural estrogens?
A: Not in their effect as replacement hormones. The terms are somewhat misleading. They make it sound as if "natural" estrogen is the kind normally found in a woman's body and "synthetic" is something made in a laboratory. Actually, the "natural" estrogen women have in their bodies can not be used medically because it is not easily absorbed into the bloodstream, and its activity is reduced or even destroyed as the body processes it through the liver and other organs. There are some so-called natural estrogens uncommonly used in treatment (for example, micronized estradiol and esterified estradiol) that are manufactured from chemicals so that they are chemically identical to human estrogen. Synthetic estrogens such as ethinyl estradiol and quinestrol are manufactured in the laboratory and are chemically different from human estro-

gen, but mimic its effect in the body. Finally, one of the most commonly used estrogens, conjugated equine estrogen, comes from the urine of pregnant mares. It has been modified in the laboratory so that your body can effectively metabolize it and put it to use.

Q: What are the most common side effects of HRT?

A: Before getting into the details, it is a good idea to repeat a basic rule about side effects: No one will experience every side effect reported for a particular drug. A doctor who prescribes a new medication has an obligation to let you know what to expect, both good and bad. This means informing you of all the effects that have been reported by a certain number of people who have taken that medicine. Some people have had several; some people none. Certain individuals are quite susceptible to certain kinds of side effects (stomach upsets, for example, or skin rashes) while others seem to be quite immune. You might have one side effect and no others, or you might have several. And, of course, you might have a mild version or a severe one. Doctors cannot predict; all they can say is "a lot of people who take this medicine get headaches" or "very few of my patients have complained of nausea." It is important to remember that many side effects are temporary when you begin a new treatment, and that others can be reduced or eliminated by changing dosages, the form of the medicine taken, or the treatment schedule.

Specifically, common untoward symptoms that have been reported with HRT include sensitivities to dyes, binders, or oils used in the medicine; headaches; tiredness; itching; rash; difficulty sleeping or concentrating; a form of PMS; mood changes; nausea; and a tendency toward blood clots. Hormone replacement that is high in progestin may produce bloating, weight gain, fluid retention, and depression. Some women report that when they first started taking hormones, they had some of the symptoms of early pregnancy, including bloating, breast tenderness, morning sickness, and slight mood changes. These seem to either go away on their own after a few months or can be relieved by changing the dosage.

Q: What are the most serious side effects of HRT?
A: Most of the widely publicized serious side effects were associated with earlier, high-dose, estrogen-only forms of hormone therapy and are no longer a real problem. These included abnormal clotting, strokes, and the long-term increased risks of breast and endometrial cancer. Monthly menstrual-type bleeding is a common result of hormone therapy that many women consider the most undesirable side effect.

Q: Can anything be done about the monthly bleeding that occurs with HRT?
A: The newer continuous dose regimens generally limit monthly bleeding, which is actually more like spotting, to the first three months or

so of treatment. After that, only a few women still have the problem. Unfortunately, it tends to be unpredictable, coming and going without warning, which some women find unacceptable. Your doctor may be able to find a regimen that eliminates the problem for you.

If you are one of the very small minority of women who have rather heavy bleeding with cramps and other menstrual complaints, you can take one of the pain relievers that contains prostaglandin inhibitors, such as ibuprofen. Some adjustments in dosage may help. It is important that you discuss this fully with your doctor.

Q: Does HRT make you gain weight?
A: This is a controversy that is probably not going to go away easily. Much has been written and said about it, but there does not seem to be one single, definitive, persuasive scientific study on one side or the other. Part of the problem is that women of menopausal age tend to gain some weight whether they are taking hormones or not, but the gain has been attributed to hormones by those who are on HRT. What does seem to be fairly widely accepted is that if there is any weight gain, it is not much—no more than five pounds on average. Proper diet and exercise can control this whether the cause is middle age, menopause, or hormones.

Q: Does HRT prevent premature menopause?
A: No, but it can have some effect in controlling it, just as HRT "corrects" the drop in estrogen

that comes from normal menopause. The most significant effect is in counteracting the early loss of fertility from premature menopause (before age forty). One study showed that about a third of women with this problem could be helped to become pregnant through a combination of HRT, in-vitro fertilization, and egg donation.

Q: Are there particular reasons why I shouldn't take HRT?
A: You should not take it if you smoke, because of the increased risk of heart attack among women smokers. Other conditions that rule out HRT are pregnancy, endometriosis, recent endometrial or breast cancer, active liver disease, hypertension, or any blood clotting disorder.

Q: When should I start taking HRT?
A: This depends on whether you want to use HRT for menopausal symptoms or for long-term health protection. If for symptoms, you should begin as soon as you see the first signs of menopause. For long-term protection, the ideal time to start is as you approach menopause, before you start to experience symptoms.

Q: How long will I have to take hormones?
A: For hot flashes, you might take them from several months to a year, including a tapering-off period. For long-term benefit, it is generally agreed that you need a minimum of ten years but that continued lifetime treatment is ideal.

This will be discussed in greater detail in Chapter 6.

Q: What tests should be done before HRT is given?
A: Most physicians recommend a mammogram if you have not had one for three years or if you have a family history of any form of breast disease. Any woman with a family history of ovarian cancer should have an ultrasound examination; many doctors recommend that women at risk of this cancer should have ultrasound exams on a regular basis. Some physicians take hormone profiles, but the general consensus is that these are not very significant, except in diagnosing premature menopause in women under forty who have what appear to be menopausal symptoms. In some cases, a study of the levels and kinds of lipids in the bloodstream can be helpful in making later comparisons to assess the effect of HRT on cardiovascular health, but such studies rarely make any difference in the doctor's recommendations about HRT. A woman who has had abnormal bleeding—heavy flow or bleeding between periods or after intercourse—may need an endometrial biopsy. Most doctors do not do expensive bone scans for signs of osteoporosis except for women who have high risk factors. These include early menopause, low weight for your height, a family history of osteoporosis, sedentary lifestyle, alcohol abuse, cigarette smoking, high caffeine intake, and other circumstances including steroid therapy and hyperthyroidism.

SIX

Risks and Myths

CASE STUDY

As a 54-year-old medical writer, Gwen knew more than most women about the purported risks and benefits of HRT when she visited her gynecologist with several menopause-related complaints, including mood swings and chronic hot flashes. Factors in her personal and family medical history dissuaded her gynecologist from recommending the use of hormone replacement to alleviate her symptoms.

"My grandmother died from breast cancer and I have mild fibrocystic breast disease, and that was all she needed to know," Gwen said.

"She explained that HRT could dramatically increase my risk of breast cancer, and she refused to back down on the issue. I told her that I was aware of all my options, including alternative therapies, and realized the potential danger of hormone replacement, but that I didn't think it was serious enough to stop me from trying estrogen. For me, the benefits outweighed the risks. But she disagreed. She was like a rock."

Gwen did a little more research on HRT, and became even more convinced that she was a suitable candidate. She approached her gynecologist one last time with her request, but could not sway her doctor's opinion.

Gwen came to me for a second opinion. I examined her medical history and talked with her at length about her decision. I also explained to her that some studies suggested that HRT could increase her risk of certain health problems. She decided that the risks were acceptable.

I performed a mammogram and a Pap smear on Gwen, and prescribed a very low-dose estrogen tablet with the understanding that I would consider increasing the dosage only if Gwen did not find relief.

"The low-dose therapy worked well," Gwen said later. "My hormone levels and overall health are being closely monitored, and I feel good about my decision."

According to the medical literature, only about one-third of all menopausal women try HRT, compared to one-half of all female doctors of menopausal age. What do we make of the disparity between these two statistics? Is the fact that so many female doctors are pro-HRT a ringing endorsement of estrogen as a risk-free wonder drug? They presumably have access to the most reliable information and the skill necessary to interpret it. If that is the case, what about the other 50 percent of female doctors who do not use it? What do they know that the first group does not? Part of the answer can be explained by the fact that a lot of the current information regarding HRT is conflicting, meaning that several similar studies have come to different conclusions. These and other considerations about hormone replacement often make decision-making difficult, but not impossible. The first step is to find a physician who is knowledgeable and experienced in the area of female reproductive health and the benefits and risks of HRT (see Chapter 9). Your doctor's expertise and your own willingness to play an active role in your health care can make the process easier.

A lack of information on the part of your doctor is a potential factor that may confound a woman's attempt to get at the truth about HRT. As you have seen in the first two chapters of this book, the basic issue of female endocrinology and female reproductive health—particularly the changes that take place during and after menopause—is a very complex subject. Not every general practitioner or gynecologist has the time or the motivation to keep up with every new research study or advance in treatment. That may be one reason why two-thirds of menopausal women in one recent survey had never even discussed hormone replacement with their physicians. The fact that three-fourths of these same women said that they would probably have tried HRT if their doctors had recommended it points out the importance of finding the right doctor and may also say something about the uncritical fashion in which some women accept their doctor's opinions without doing everything they can to research the issue for themselves.

You should always use your intelligence and basic common sense in evaluating information about HRT, especially when it comes to you from sources other than your doctor. If you are inclined to look at scientific studies, which are relatively easy to access through your local or academic library and can be searched using on-line computer programs such as MEDLINE (see Chapter 9), pay more attention to prestigious journals such as the *Journal of the American Medical Association (JAMA)*, the *New England Journal of Medicine*, or *Nature*. Studies conducted at reputable research facilities are usually more important than those conducted by scientists who lack the support of a recognized granting body such as the National Institutes of Health or the American Cancer Society. Popular health and news magazines, and even your daily newspaper, often report the findings of major HRT studies and occasionally carry other related stories.

Keep in mind that a lot of information about women's hormones refers to the average woman, or to groups with particularly high or low risk factors. You may or may not fall into these specific categories, and that could influence whether or not HRT is right for you. Remember: HRT does not carry the same amount of risk for everyone. Every piece of information you receive should be put into the context of your life, your

family history, your symptoms, needs, and
health goals.

In this chapter we will discuss the risks and
benefits of HRT, common misinformation or mis-
conceptions, and how you can decide if HRT is
right for you.

**Q: I've heard so many conflicting stories regarding
HRT and cancer risk that I don't know whom
to believe anymore. Does anyone know the
truth?**

A: The degree of increased cancer risk for women
on HRT depends on whom you talk to. Every
study, it seems, reaches a different conclusion,
which makes it difficult for doctors to give their
patients an informed opinion.

For example, a study recently reported in the
Journal of Epidemiology compared 3,130 postmenopausal women diagnosed with breast cancer
and 3,698 healthy postmenopausal women, and
concluded that HRT was not linked with a breast
cancer risk in women who had at some time used
the treatment. Researchers also reported no clear
increase among the small number of patients
who had taken HRT for fifteen years or longer.

A separate study conducted at the Fred Hutch-
inson Cancer Research Center in Seattle, Washington, compared 537 middle-aged female
patients with breast cancer and 492 randomly se-
lected women with no history of breast cancer.
Menopausal hormones of some type had been
used by 57.6 percent of the women with breast
cancer and by 61 percent of the comparison
group. Compared with nonusers of menopausal

hormones, those who used a combination of estrogen/progestin HRT for eight years had what appeared to be a reduced risk of breast cancer. But the researchers stated that since the use of combined estrogen and progestin is relatively new, future studies are necessary to determine whether breast cancer incidence changes after many years of use.

The American Cancer Society also failed to find a causative link between HRT and breast cancer. Researchers there followed more than 400,000 women from 1982 to 1992, and concluded that taking estrogen for ten years did not increase a woman's risk of dying from breast cancer.

But many other studies tell a different story. One analysis involving more than 69,000 female nurses concluded that the use of hormone supplements for more than five years increases a woman's risk of breast cancer by around 50 percent. And the risk appears to be even greater for older women, with a 70 percent increase for women ages sixty to sixty-four. This study also concludes that the use of combined supplements (such as estrogen and progestin) does not reduce either the incidence of breast cancer or its mortality rate, as many researchers had hoped. Among current users, the risk rises with five or more years of use.

The National Cancer Institute, which has been analyzing the possible increase of cancer risk among HRT patients for some time, reports conflicting results. In one NCI study, postmenopausal women who had taken estrogen for twenty years or more had a 50 percent increase in cancer risk compared with those who had not taken it.

In another study of 23,000 Swedish women who took estrogen alone or in combination with progestin, researchers found a 10 percent higher incidence of breast cancer than expected. A more detailed analysis of the women who developed breast cancer and a random sample of those who did not develop the disease showed that the risk increased to 70 percent compared with the expected level among women who used the hormones for nine or more years. Again, this risk did not seem to be affected by the addition of progestin.

As you can see, there is no simple answer to this question. A great many factors are involved in determining a potential increase in breast cancer risk, including family history, the type of hormones you are taking (estrogen alone seems to result in a higher risk than when used in combination with progestin, though even that does not appear to be absolute), the amount of hormones you are taking (higher doses pose a greater risk), and the length of time you have been on HRT.

The risk of breast cancer is and should be a serious concern for any woman considering HRT, but it should not automatically preclude you from using this treatment. Conduct your own research and talk at length with your doctor regarding your individual benefit-risk ratio before making your final decision.

An article in a recent issue of *Obstetrics and Gynecology* put the issue into perspective by noting that in a hypothetical group of ten thousand women, after twenty-five years of estrogen use, the increased risk of death from breast cancer would be 21 percent. But the same group of women would see a 48 percent decrease in death risk from heart disease, and a 49 percent decrease in osteoporosis-related hip fractures. The authors that concluded that the health benefits of postmenopausal HRT exceed the health risks incurred.

Q: Could you give me a little more information regarding breast cancer, specific risk factors, and what I can do to help prevent this disease? Although I have not reached menopause yet, I want to do all I can to help myself before it is time for me to decide whether I should consider HRT.

A: Yours is a good question. Many women are unaware that certain types of breast cancer appear to be caused by lifestyle and therefore are preventable.

Before we talk risk factors and prevention, a little statistical information: Breast cancer is the second most common form of cancer among women worldwide, and the most common type among women living in developed countries. By the turn of the century, researchers predict that breast cancer will account for more than 500,000 deaths annually.

Heredity is one of the biggest risk factors for

breast cancer. A family history of the disease increases the likelihood that a woman will develop breast cancer sometime in her life. Studies show the risk of breast cancer to be two to three times higher for women with an affected first-degree relative, such as a mother or sister, and less than twice as high with an affected second-degree relative, such as a cousin.

Other risk factors include the use of hormones (especially estrogen), sociodemographics (women in higher social classes tend to have a higher rate of incidence compared to women of lower classes), and diet, especially the intake of dietary fat. More than twenty studies on laboratory mice show that a high-fat diet increases the frequency and reduces the time before the occurrence of breast cancers.

Lifestyle can also increase a woman's risk of breast cancer, but these factors are the easiest to correct. Cancer specialists advise the following.

- Exercise regularly. Physical activity in adolescence and young adulthood has been shown in clinical studies to reduce the risk of breast cancer in pre- and perimenopausal women. Some researchers speculate that this is related to the effects of exercise on hormones.

- Avoid alcohol. Just two to three drinks a day can increase a woman's risk of breast cancer by nearly 50 percent, compared to nondrinkers. Again, this increase in risk may be hormonally connected.

- Quit smoking. Though some studies have shown a reduction in risk among women who smoke, most suggest that smoking actually increases your risk. It is also bad for your lungs and heart.

- Eat a more nutritious diet. This means a reduction in dietary fat and sodium, and an increase in dietary fiber.

- Avoid certain environmental exposures, such as pesticides. Scientists are still debating just how much of an impact on risk these factors have, but it is better to be safe than sorry while additional research is being conducted.

Q: **How exactly does estrogen affect the development of breast cancer?**

A: That is a question scientists have been trying to answer for decades. And they are still trying. Every research breakthrough seems to pose more questions than it answers.

There is no evidence suggesting a direct causative relationship between HRT and the onset of breast cancer. As a result, some researchers theorize that menopausal hormones may help facilitate the development of cancer in cells that have already been sensitized by other factors, such as diet, the environment, or genetics.

The genetic connection is especially interesting in light of the discovery of so-called "susceptibility" genes. In most cases, a woman with such a gene will not develop breast cancer until something occurs on a cellular level to "turn on" the affected gene and trigger the onset of cancer. At this point, no one has pinpointed the exact cellular mechanism which may trigger cancer in this way.

Q: Is it true that researchers have discovered a gene that triggers breast cancer?

A: Yes. Scientists have isolated a particularly strong susceptibility gene for breast cancer called BRCA1, though other susceptibility genes are also known or suspected. It is estimated that one in three hundred women carry the BRCA1 gene, which is implicated in about 4 percent of breast cancers in all age groups, and 25 percent of those diagnosed before age forty. Women who carry BRCA1 have an 85 percent chance of developing breast cancer by the age of eighty, and more than half will develop the disease before age fifty.

The discovery of this gene means that one day researchers may discover a way to "switch it off," dramatically reducing the risk of breast cancer in women who carry it. In addition, women who are found to carry the gene are able to receive more thorough health examinations in hopes of catching the disease earlier, should it occur at all.

Q: I've heard that the risk of breast cancer is higher among slender women using HRT than among those who are heavier. Is this true?

A: It appears so. In a recent issue of the *Journal*

of the American Medical Association, researchers at Ohio State University reviewed clinical evidence that suggested a 70 percent increase in breast cancer risk associated with HRT in lean, postmenopausal women. Based on this finding, the researchers suggested additional studies regarding the impact of ERT on this particular subgroup.

Q: Does pregnancy reduce a woman's risk of developing breast cancer?
A: Studies in mice suggest that early full-term pregnancy removes what are known as "susceptible proliferating cells" from the breasts. Carcinogens produced fewer breast tumors in mice that underwent early pregnancy compared to those that did not.

This may be good news for mice, but it is of less importance to us, until relevant human studies can establish the same link.

Q: Should I get a mammogram before I agree to HRT?
A: Yes. In fact, most doctors will automatically suggest a pretreatment mammogram to detect any potentially dangerous lumps or lesions, and to provide a baseline X ray for future comparison.

Once you have started HRT, you should examine your breasts each month and note any new lumps or changes in appearance. Self-exams can be helpful in bringing changes to the attention of your doctor, but they should not be relied upon. You must get an annual breast exam and complete physical from your doctor to catch problems in their early, treatable stages.

Q: **My best friend is supposed to be on HRT, but has yet to get her prescription filled because she's afraid of getting breast cancer. Is fear-based noncompliance a common problem among women who receive HRT?**

A: Yes, it is a very big problem. According to some medical analysts, as many as 50 percent of women with a prescription for HRT still are not taking the drug after more than a year—and many never even get their prescriptions filled.

Like your friend, most of these noncompliant women are reluctant to receive HRT because of fear of breast cancer and other medical complications. Others start HRT then stop abruptly because they cannot tolerate the side effects.

Q: **Does HRT increase a woman's risk of endometrial cancer?**

A: The answer is yes, but with qualifications.

Cancer of the endometrium—the inner lining of the uterus—is the nation's most common cancer of the reproductive tract, affecting one in every one thousand women. When caught in precancerous stages, it can be treated without radical surgery, and the cure rate is virtually 100 percent.

Postmenopausal women who have not had a hysterectomy and who take unopposed estrogen (without progestogen) are from two to thirteen times more likely to develop endometrial cancer than those who do not take estrogen. In other words, ten to twenty out of every thousand women who have taken estrogen alone will develop endometrial cancer, compared to one in one thousand nonusers.

The fact is that more than 99 percent of post-menopausal estrogen users do not develop endometrial cancer. Further, most endometrial cancers associated with estrogen use are of the less aggressive types, and are typically caught in the early stages because women on estrogen therapy get more frequent medical checkups and closer monitoring.

Researchers also report that women taking a combination of estrogen and progestogen have a risk of endometrial cancer that is actually lower than that of women who take no hormones at all. This is because progesterone causes the endometrium to slough away every month.

Because of the increased risk of cancer associated with the use of estrogen, the Food and Drug Administration (FDA) requires that an informative brochure be included with each estrogen prescription. The brochure reports that the risk of endometrial cancer increases with estrogen use according to dosage strength and duration.

Q: How effectively does HRT protect women from coronary heart disease?

A: More than thirty-two clinical studies have been conducted on the effects of HRT on female cardiac health, and nearly all of them concluded that protection from heart disease is one of the most important long-term benefits of HRT. (Estrogen has no protective effect on male hearts because they lack the proper hormone receptors.)

An estimated 25 percent of estrogen's protective ability comes from reducing harmful cholesterol levels in the blood. It also has positive effects on just about every aspect of the cardiovascular system, from the blood vessels to the heart itself.

Most cardiovascular studies involved unopposed estrogen, but more recent analysis at Brigham and Women's Hospital in Boston suggests that a combination of estrogen and progestin works equally well at protecting the heart while also reducing the risk of endometrial cancer. The finding was based on up to sixteen years of follow-up in 59,337 women who were between the ages of thirty and fifty-five at baseline.

Q: I had a heart attack a few years ago, and recovered quite well. Does my history of heart disease mean that HRT won't benefit my heart in the future?

A: No. Believe it or not, some studies have found that the beneficial effects of estrogen on the heart are actually stronger in women who have existing coronary heart disease.

In one study, researchers spent ten years following one thousand women who were diagnosed with extreme coronary heart disease. Those who received estrogen had an 84 percent reduction in their risk of recurrent disease, and 97 percent were still alive at the end of the study.

Q: I had a tumor removed from my cervix when I was in my mid-twenties. Could going on HRT to manage my menopause symptoms cause this type of cancer to return?

A: No. Cancers of the vulva or cervix are not hormone dependent (as are breast and uterine cancer), so there is no reason to think that HRT will have any impact on your condition.

Q: Can HRT increase a woman's risk of venous thrombosis?

A: Yes. Venous thrombosis, in which blood clots form in the veins of the legs and elsewhere, has been associated in numerous studies with the use of estrogen, most often with oral contraceptives. But two recent British studies tackled the question of whether HRT poses an increased risk among menopausal and postmenopausal women and found an increase—about three to four times higher for HRT users than nonusers. A history of blood clots may compound your risk.

Women with a history of thrombosis who still want to try HRT should consider an estrogen patch or cream rather than an oral supplement. Studies show less of a clotting risk from these delivery systems, though you should still have your blood monitored frequently to detect any changes in anticlotting factors.

Q: Can HRT really help me live longer?
A: HRT may help you live longer by reducing your risk of certain medical conditions known to kill women at an earlier age, such as heart disease, osteoporosis, Alzheimer's disease, and perhaps even stroke.

A review of clinical studies concluded that women on HRT can expect a four-year increase in life expectancy—and even more if they take especially good care of their health.

Q: My best friend told me that my high cholesterol level could increase my risk of developing gallstones if I go on HRT. Is this true?
A: Yes. Clinical studies have found that estrogen—with or without progesterone—can result in a twofold increase in gallbladder stones made of cholesterol.

This is because estrogen tends to force cholesterol in the liver into bile for elimination. Bile collects in the gallbladder, which eventually dumps it into the intestine so it can be eliminated in our stool. Unfortunately, the greater the concentration of cholesterol in the bile, the greater the chances it will eventually form painful stones.

If you would still like to receive HRT, talk to your doctor about using an estrogen patch rather than pills. There is a good chance it will decrease estrogen's effect on the liver and reduce your risk of gallbladder stones.

Q: **My doctor expressed concern over the fact that I have a mild form of liver disease when I brought up the issue of HRT. Could my condition prevent me from going on hormones?**

A: Probably not. There is no clinical evidence that estrogen therapy influences liver disease, so your doctor was probably just being cautious.

But you should be wary of estrogen in pill form. Oral estrogen is metabolized by the liver and tends to accumulate there. For healthy women, this poses few problems. But for women with pre-existing liver disease, the high level of hormones could become toxic, or put unwanted stress on an already overworked and diseased organ. Common causes of liver disease include alcohol abuse and hepatitis.

Because of your condition, your doctor will probably suggest an alternative form of delivery, such as an estrogen patch or implant. These methods pump estrogen directly into the bloodstream, bypassing the liver and intestinal tract.

Q: **I've been taking medication for moderate hypertension for nearly fifteen years. Is this something my doctor needs to know when we discuss HRT?**

A: Yes. An estimated one in twenty women who take oral estrogen tablets experience an increase in blood pressure because of the release of two special enzymes, renin and angiotensin. This can be potentially dangerous for women with high blood pressure because a sudden increase in pressure can cause serious medical complications.

If you really want to try HRT, consider a non-oral method of delivery, such as an estrogen patch or cream. They pose far less risk when it comes to hypertension.

Q: With all the conflicting information, and new data being released almost daily, how can any woman make an informed decision regarding the use of HRT? Is there a way to simplify this procedure?

A: The use of HRT is not a decision that should be made lightly or in haste. There are a lot benefits but there are a lot of potential risks as well.

Many doctors encourage their patients to work through the decision by creating an individualized chart that evaluates all of the important factors in the use of HRT. For some women, this chart is rather simple; for others, it is quite detailed and complicated. But in the end, you and your doctor will be able to make a very informed decision that takes into equal consideration your medical history and current needs.

The first part of your chart should detail the specific reasons why you want to try HRT. For most women, it is to ease the symptoms of menopause, though your reasons may be different. A good doctor will require a very valid reason for considering this treatment option.

Once you have determined the reason you want to try HRT, you and your doctor should discuss and write down any and all relevant medical conditions that might be affected by the use of HRT. These include, but are not limited to, the presence of noneradicated endometrial cancer, the presence or history of breast cancer, active thrombosis, chronic liver or kidney disease, and pregnancy.

The presence of some medical conditions means that you should, under no circumstances, receive HRT. At this point, you should discuss alternative treatment options with your physician. If you have other conditions, depending on severity and other factors, the possibility of HRT may be open to discussion and evaluation. It is during this phase that you should listen very closely to your doctor's advice. If you decide to pursue HRT against his recommendations, he may ask you to sign a waiver that absolves him of responsibility should adverse side effects develop.

If you have no medical conditions that HRT is thought to adversely affect, you and your doctor should then discuss your family's medical history, such as a history of breast cancer in distant relatives, or past history of thromboembolism and moderate endometriosis.

If you have none of these, you may be a good candidate for HRT. If you have one or two, then you and your doctor must weigh present and future benefits against potential risks. Some of these considerations carry greater weight than others, and will influence many factors should you decide to proceed, including when HRT should be started, the size of the dose you will receive, and the duration of treatment.

If you have any questions after you have completed the chart, or you are still unsure whether HRT is right for you, do not hesitate to talk more with your doctor. Admit your concerns and ask for more guidance in making this important decision. HRT has many benefits, but it is not for everyone and the decision to try it should not be made without thorough consideration.

Q: My doctor recently mentioned that estrogen appears to have a beneficial effect on Alzheimer's disease. Is this true?

A: Preliminary studies suggest it is, but do not look for an estrogen-based Alzheimer's cure just yet. Quite a bit more work remains to be done before doctors will be able to say with certainty that estrogen is the "magic bullet" they have been looking for.

Still, the work done so far is promising. In one British study, researchers followed one thousand elderly women for five years. The 156 women who reported taking estrogen demonstrated a significantly lower risk of developing Alzheimer's disease than those who didn't—5.8 percent compared to 16.3 percent. In addition, women with Alzheimer's disease who had used estrogen demonstrated symptoms much later than those who did not use estrogen.

In another study conducted at the University of Southern California, researchers followed more than nine thousand postmenopausal women for several years. They found that those who received long-term estrogen lived far longer than those who did not receive the hormone—and that at the time of their deaths, the women on estrogen had a 40 percent lower incidence of Alzheimer's disease.

Researchers still have a lot of work ahead of them, but the implications of these preliminary studies are intriguing. Estrogen may improve memory and lower the risk of Alzheimer's disease in the population most at risk—older women. It is hoped that future research will also shed light on how estrogen affects the brain, as well as the developmental path of Alzheimer's disease and other forms of senile dementia.

Q: I'm a pretty heavy smoker. Does this pose any additional hazards if I receive HRT?
A: It has long been established that high-dose oral contraceptives can increase clotting factors in the blood and that smoking can exacerbate this problem, leading to the formation of potentially dangerous blood clots in the heart. But this does not occur with the type of hormones used in HRT. In fact, they tend to have the opposite effect by decreasing clot formation.

But it is wrong to think that HRT will fix all the problems that result from smoking. Just the opposite is true. Women who smoke tend to have lower blood levels of estrogen than those who do not smoke, and there is some evidence that smoking increases the breakdown of estrogen in the liver. In addition, smoking tends to stimulate the production of adrenal hormones that oppose the effects of estrogen.

All of these are very good reasons to stop smoking if you are considering HRT. You should also consider the harmful effects smoking has on your lungs, heart, and other body systems.

Q: I have a history of benign fibroid tumors of the uterus. Will HRT cause a flare-up of this condition once I reach menopause?

A: Probably not. Even though estrogen is the cause of most benign fibroid tumors of the uterus in premenopausal women, there is very little evidence that the traditional doses of hormones used in HRT will cause a recurrence.

Be aware that some forms of fibroid tumors can grow into the endometrial cavity, and cause heavy bleeding with the use of HRT. In most cases, these growths cannot be detected without an ultrasound. If you experience heavy bleeding once you start HRT, consult your physician at once. He will probably give you two options: cease HRT, or have the fibroids surgically removed.

Q: My doctor wants to prescribe progesterone for my menopause-related hot flashes. Isn't it estrogen that I need?

A: Estrogen has been used for decades to ease the most common symptoms of menopause, including hot flashes. But recent research now suggests that progesterone may work equally well without the side effects commonly associated with estrogen. Nonetheless, estrogen remains the most commonly prescribed hormone supplement in the United States.

Progesterone is a hormone with an increasingly wide range of uses, though it is especially beneficial to menopausal women in that it effectively reduces hot flashes in up to 80 percent of the women who use it. It also works well in the prevention or treatment of osteoporosis, endometrial cancer, and other medical problems such as fluid retention.

Side effects associated with progesterone therapy include depression and mood swings, breast tenderness or enlargement, an increase in appetite (by affecting blood sugar levels), headaches, and possible adverse changes in blood lipid levels.

Any side effects should be discussed at once with your physician. Most can be eliminated with a simple dosage adjustment or change in lifestyle.

Q: Because the jury is still out regarding HRT and breast cancer risk, I'd like to try a more natural approach to treating my menopause symptoms, specifically hot flashes and vaginal dryness. Any recommendations?

A: Dr. Andrew Weil, one of the world's most respected authorities on natural medicine, suggests the following herbal concoction for hot flashes:

At a health food store, get capsules of dong quai chaste tree (Vitex agnus-castus) and damiana (Turnera diffusa). Take two capsules of each around noon each day. Continue until your hot flashes disappear, then gradually cut the dose until you do not need it anymore.

As for vaginal dryness, you might want to try one of the many natural, over-the-counter vaginal lubricants currently available. Most are water soluble and completely safe when used as directed.

Q: **You've mentioned a lot of potentially serious side effects regarding the use of HRT. What about minor side effects?**

A: There can be plenty of those, too. Every woman's reaction to HRT is unique. Some women never have a single problem, while others experience an abundance of aggravating ailments.

The most common side effects associated with HRT include nausea, bloating, fluid retention, irritability, breast tenderness, and an unwanted increase in breast size. In addition, women who suffer from chronic headaches may experience an increase in number and severity, though most headache sufferers report greater relief after starting hormone therapy.

Most of these problems disappear once the body adjusts to HRT. But some women find the problems so difficult to tolerate that they ask their doctors to stop the treatment. In cases such as these, the answer often lies in changing brands, adjusting hormone levels—or encouraging the patient to alter her lifestyle. High doses of caffeine, for example, can increase breast tenderness among women on HRT. A high salt intake and lack of exercise can also exacerbate certain problems such as fluid retention.

SEVEN

Who Takes HRT?

CASE STUDY

Jeanne first came to me with a list of symptoms that had her puzzled. Her periods had become heavier and irregular, and she was starting to experience occasional hot flashes and vaginal dryness that made sex with her husband somewhat painful.

"At first, I thought that it might have something to do with the new exercise regimen I had started," she said. "But the problems continued even when I cut back. That's when I thought I should see a doctor."

I gave Jeanne a thorough examination, including a blood test, and determined that she was perimenopausal, or approaching menopause. "But I'm only forty-seven," she said. "I shouldn't be going through change of life for another ten years."

I explained that onset of menopause at age forty-seven was completely normal. I told Jeanne that the symptoms that she was experiencing were the result of a small but measurable decrease in hormone production. I discussed various treatment approaches with her and suggested an ultra-low-dose contraceptive pill to alleviate her menopausal symptoms.

After about three or four weeks, Jeanne reported that her hot flashes had decreased in frequency and intensity, and sex was no longer uncomfortable. Her periods also became more regular again.

"To me, menopause meant old age, and I don't think of myself as old," Jeanne said. "It wasn't something I really thought about, so I was surprised when I found myself entering the first stages of it."

When a woman over forty years old has night sweats and hot flashes, even if she has no other symptoms (such as vaginal dryness), a doctor has no difficulty making a diagnosis of menopause. In fact, many women make the diagnosis themselves. But like Jeanne, women who believe they are too young to be going through the "change of life" may be surprised at their doctor's findings. What may be even more surprising is that HRT is not limited to menopausal or postmenopausal women. Those who are just beginning to enter this stage of their lives can also benefit from HRT, as well as women with premature menopause (before age forty) and amenorrhea, polycystic ovaries, and even Alzheimer's disease, although this use is still experimental.

Who, then, is the woman who takes HRT? As we have just seen, she may be either perimenopausal, menopausal, or postmenopausal. She is likely to be white, well-educated, and in a higher socioeconomic bracket. Sadly, working class or poor women in other ethnic groups may have less access to health care and thus may not even be aware of HRT as a treatment option. The HRT user also tends to be well informed about such issues as estrogen deficiency and its role in menopause. She is therefore more likely to use sound judgment regarding HRT as an appropriate option for her. Studies show that she is also more likely to see a female gynecologist and to live on the West Coast compared with the East Coast.

We also know the characteristics of the woman whom HRT will probably benefit most. She may have been taking corticosteroids or thyroxine; have heart disease, diabetes, or a family history of high blood lipids; be at risk for or already have osteoporosis; or she may have had her uterus or ovaries removed before she reached menopause. Or, she may simply be experiencing disruptive or uncomfortable symptoms of menopause such as hot flashes and vaginal dryness. The presence of any of these conditions is a good reason to consider HRT therapy, and for many of them, clinical evidence exists to prove HRT's efficacy.

This chapter will discuss the characteristics of the HRT user and examine some of the demographic patterns seen in its use.

Q: How many women have menopausal symptoms severe enough to use HRT?

A: It is estimated that about 75 percent of menopausal women in America have hot flashes. But only 10 percent to 15 percent have symptoms severe enough to make them visit a doctor. A significant factor is how long the hot flashes last. Many women will put up with them if they do not go on too long. On average, they are more frequent during the first two years after menopause, then taper off or stop. About 85 percent of women have hot flashes for more than a year, and 20 percent to 50 percent have them for up to five years. Most women seem to have hot flashes between 6 a.m. and 8 a.m. and again between 6 p.m. and 10 p.m. This means the discomfort and inconvenience are limited to nonworking hours and to periods when a woman can avoid the embarrassment of being around other people if she prefers, which may make treatment seem unnecessary. But keep in mind that HRT is prescribed not just for such symptoms, but also for the prevention of certain health risks that come with the decline in estrogen.

Q: How many women take HRT?

A: The exact number is not really known. There are about 40 million women in this country over age forty-five. Only about a third of all menopausal women try HRT, or about 13 million. The numbers are very different in other countries; in Great Britain, for example, only 12 percent of menopausal women take hormones. In coming years, the numbers will probably increase. The total number of menopausal women in the United States is expected to reach 60 million within ten years.

Q: Do women doctors take HRT more than other women?

A: Yes. One survey of more than a thousand female doctors age forty-five to sixty-five showed that half had tried HRT and 41 percent still use it.

Q: Women—like my mother, for instance—used to go through menopause without medication. Why has HRT become such an urgent, talked-about subject?

A: The significant words in your question are "go through" menopause. That is what many women did, with a great deal of unnecessary suffering. Today, with a great variety of treatments including—but not limited to—hormone replacement, you do not have to suffer menopausal symptoms. Furthermore, many of those women who survived the most difficult period later suffered serious illnesses because of estrogen deficiency. The issue is a frequent topic today because we now have a better understanding of a woman's need for hormones and how she can safely meet those needs; we have better ways of diagnosing and treating hormonal imbalances; and we have a population of women who are better informed and more concerned about participating in their own health maintenance and care. Finally, the extraordinary fact is that today a woman who reaches fifty has an average life expectancy of eighty-five. That means she will have many more postmenopausal years in her life than women of your mother's or her mother's generation. So she spends a longer time at risk for certain postmenopausal diseases.

Q: **What are some of the reasons women don't take HRT even when their doctors recommend it?**
A: Fears, often based on misunderstanding or lack of information, play an important role. A major problem seems to be that many women do not discuss HRT with their doctors, apparently because their doctors do not bring it up. One survey of a group of postmenopausal women who had never taken HRT showed that almost two-thirds (64 percent) had never discussed it with their physicians. Three-fourths of those women said that if their doctors had recommended it, they would probably have tried it. Women are particularly open to the possibility of taking HRT if they have a specific reason, such as a definite diagnosis of osteoporosis. Much also depends on whether a woman is more concerned about just adding years to her life or whether she is interested in avoiding some of the more troubling problems of age—hip fractures being an important example. It is striking that about 20 percent of women in one survey said they absolutely would not take HRT because they did not want to continue—or resume—menstruation.

Q: **Who are the women who need HRT the most?**
A: First, women who have a high specific risk, meaning those who have been taking corticosteroid drugs; those on long-term thyroid hormone; those with known coronary disease, diabetes mellitus, or familial hyperlipidemia; and those who have had a premenopausal hysterectomy or oophorectomy. That last group is rather large: It is estimated that by age sixty, one-third of all American women have had a hysterectomy; the estimate, according to some, is as high as 58 percent. Other candidates include women who are suffering the more troublesome symptoms of menopause, including hot flashes and vaginal dryness with pain during intercourse, for example, and those who are at high risk for osteoporosis. Unfortunately, according to the National Osteoporosis Society, fewer than one in five women who should take HRT do so, and many of them eventually drop out. Another showed that among three thousand women whose ovaries had been removed, 40 percent had not even been told about HRT by their physicians. Some specialists feel that HRT has such potential benefits compared to risks that any menopausal woman is a good candidate as long as she has no health reason for avoiding HRT.

For those in the above-named risk groups, there are documented benefits with HRT use. As an example, in more than one thousand women with extreme coronary artery disease, an 84 percent reduction in their risk of recurrent disease was seen among those who received estrogen, and at the end of the ten-year study, 97 percent of the women were still alive. Estrogen-treated women were also found to have half the heart disease risk of women who did not receive treatment in the Nurses' Health Study, which followed over 48,000 postmenopausal nurses for ten years. When used as a preventive measure against osteoporosis, HRT has also been shown to reduce or stop the rate of bone loss and cut the occurrence of hip fractures in half. In the Framingham study, women under age seventy-five who had taken long-term estrogen therapy were found to have higher bone density than those who had not.

Q: Who are the women most likely to decide in favor of HRT?

A: The highest rates of HRT use are among women in upper socioeconomic brackets. White women are far more likely to use it than black or Mexican-American women. Users of HRT tend to be less obese, more physically active, and more highly educated than nonusers. They are more likely to have started menopause earlier than nonusers, to be mothers and to be currently married, to drink alcohol, and to have smoked at some time in their lives. They also appear to be better informed about HRT than women who do not take it. One survey showed that 90 percent of HRT users understood that estrogen deficiency is a major reason for menopause, compared with only 27 percent of nonusers.

Q: Am I more likely to be prescribed HRT if I have a woman gynecologist?

A: Yes. Study after study has shown that a female gynecologist is more likely than a male to recommend hormone therapy to her patients. You may be as much as five times more likely to receive postmenopausal HRT from a woman doctor. The female-male difference holds true for other medical specialties too, at least in certain areas. In Boston, for example, women internists were eleven times more likely to prescribe HRT than male internists. There is probably a close link between these patterns and the fact that women physicians also perform more cancer-screening tests (such as Pap smears and mammograms), suggesting that they are simply more alert to and have more positive attitudes about prevention and treatment of diseases unique to women. It was once suggested that the patients of women gynecologists were more likely to take HRT simply because women who choose to go to women doctors in the first place are more active about taking care of their health, but this has not been proved or disproved.

Q: Do my chances of getting HRT depend on where I live?

A: Yes. Women on the West Coast are three times as likely to use HRT than those on the East Coast, which suggests that West Coast physicians prescribe it more frequently.

Q: **Why do patterns of estrogen use vary so much from place to place and doctor to doctor? Isn't the decision scientific?**

A: It is far more complex than that. For example, in some areas women may put more pressure on their doctors to give them HRT. The emphasis on youth and appearance on the West Coast may explain in part why HRT use is more prevalent there than in the East. Costs may influence decisions among those who are underinsured or uninsured. Most important, there is no scientific way to decide which risks are more important. A survey of British physicians asked if even a small increase in the risk of cancer, either of the breast or uterus, would persuade them not to use estrogens, no matter how much benefit they offer in protection against heart disease. The physicians could not reach a consensus. Doctors often distinguish between what they think in principle—or as scientists—and the decisions they make about an individual patient. One survey revealed that 60 percent of physicians would consider HRT for their women patients but were actually prescribing it to less than 10 percent of those who were eligible candidates for the therapy. Another survey had these disquieting results: Doctors who did not prescribe HRT listed as a major reason their concerns that the danger of endometrial cancer outweighed the benefits of osteoporosis prevention—even though the same physicians said they understood that adding progestin in HRT reduced the endometrial cancer danger. All these things may help explain the low proportion of HRT use among women who might benefit from it.

Q: Are women more likely to be given HRT by a gynecologist than a family doctor?
A: Not according to one survey, which showed that the probability of prescribing HRT was 0.42 for gynecologists and 0.40 for family physicians—in other words, virtually no difference. The figures also mean that more than half of both kinds of doctors chose not to prescribe HRT at all.

Q: Who decides, the woman or her doctor?
A: Probably the best approach is for the doctor and patient to discuss the issue together. In this way, the patient has all the information necessary to make a rational decision, and the doctor has a thorough understanding of how the patient's concerns, fears, attitudes, preferences, and even finances might be affecting her decision. Some women, for example, are more concerned about leading a healthy life than just living a long one. Many studies have shown that women have much better medical and emotional results when they are given a choice and a role in treatment, for example, in managing ulcers and diabetes or, more significantly, deciding which kind of breast surgery to have. These findings have had so much impact that at least eighteen states have passed laws encouraging doctors to give patients all the information available about breast cancer surgery choices. Some studies have shown that about 50 percent of women who

were given such treatment choices had a positive attitude toward their decision after the treatment was completed.

Q: Do most women follow the recommendation to take HRT over a long term?

A: No. Some data suggest that half of those who start taking HRT drop out eventually. For example, a California survey of 671 women age sixty-five to ninety-four, during the period 1972 to 1991, showed that 146 of them used hormones continuously for fifteen years or more, 331 used hormones intermittently, and 194 never used HRT. A Massachusetts study showed 20 percent of patients never filled their prescriptions for hormone replacement medication. In Great Britain, 78 percent of women prescribed HRT stayed on it for a year, but only 19 percent continued for five years. The overall dropout rate in Great Britain is 80 percent.

Q: Are there other common reasons for hormone replacement besides menopause?

A: HRT is sometimes used to relieve some of the symptoms of amenorrhea (no menstrual cycles) caused by hormonal imbalance. (Amenorrhea also can be caused by malnutrition, emotional problems, and excessive dieting and/or exercise; these are not treatable with hormones.) HRT may also be used to relieve symptoms of polycystic ovaries, which include excessive body and facial hair and acne resulting from too much "male" hormone. It is being used in attempts to prevent or lessen the symptoms of Alzheimer's disease, even though the evidence that HRT is useful for this is not conclusive. One study in 1991 and 1992 in California showed that the rate of Alzheimer's disease seemed to fall in proportion to the amount of HRT women had taken, and that higher doses and longer treatment seemed to increase the effect.

Q: Do women with premature menopause ever take HRT, and does it do any good?
A: Many women who have very early menopause—before they are forty, for example—have not finished or sometimes even started their families and are deeply disturbed by the threatened loss of fertility. HRT has been reported to achieve a 35 percent success rate in helping such women become pregnant, although mostly through *in vitro* fertilization or egg donation. HRT does not suddenly make the ovaries able to produce eggs if menopause is already well underway, but it does allow women to support a pregnancy. Doses of HRT often need to be higher in younger women.

Q: Do some women have HRT in connection with cancer treatment?
A: Yes. The menstrual cycle is usually interrupted by cancer chemotherapy. HRT may be used to prevent menopause in women of reproductive years or—in older women—to avoid the symptoms of sudden "surgical" menopause.

Q: Is it true that Asian women hardly ever take HRT?

A: HRT is not as widely used in many populations—including Asian and African countries—as in America and other Western nations. Asian women's experience of and attitude toward menopause is noticeably different from the Western viewpoint. One of many studies on this subject showed, for example, that 60 percent of menopausal Canadian women report having hot flashes compared to only 20 percent of Japanese women. One theory to explain this difference is that Asian women get a lot of plant estrogen in their diet. What is not known is whether Japanese women actually have hot flashes as often as Western women but simply do not report them. In some cultures, women of mature years are greatly valued, so that they are less concerned with the emotional and psychological impact of menopause and thus are not as affected by menopausal symptoms.

EIGHT

❧

The Alternatives

CASE STUDY

Sharon, a 52-year-old bank teller, expressed interest in acupuncture as a way of alleviating her menopause symptoms, including hot flashes, mild depression, and occasional cramps. "A friend of mine has used acupuncture for years, and swears by its effectiveness," she told me during a visit. "I'd like to try it."

Sharon was quite serious in her pursuit, so I arranged for her to see a well-respected acupuncture practitioner near her home. Two months later I saw Sharon for a follow-up visit and asked her about her acupuncture treatments.

"I was a little nervous at first," she said. "The idea of being stuck with needles frightened me. But much to my amazement, the needles didn't hurt at all. More importantly, the treatments really seemed to ease my menopause symptoms. My hot flashes were less intense, my depression eased, and the cramps became less frequent.

"I'm pleased with my decision to give acupuncture a try. It made the first stages of menopause a lot easier to bear."

Several years ago, the United States government created the Office of Alternative Medicine in the National Institutes of Health. For the first time in our history, mainstream medicine officially recognized that approaches other than traditional and conventional medicine might have validity—that they at least deserved investigation, not automatic dismissal or contempt.

Among the first research projects to be funded by the new office was a grant to Columbia University's Center for Alternative Medicine for research on nonmainstream treatments for menopausal symptoms caused by estrogen deficiency. The study of a combination of twelve plant remedies used for centuries in China will be conducted by an American physiologist noted for her studies of hot flashes, an American endocrinologist, a Chinese physician, and a Chinese herbalist and certified acupuncturist.

Even for women who themselves prefer to remain within the mainstream for their health care, this is good news. It is one more demonstration of the success of the movement toward more medical options, more freedom of choice, and more participation by the individual in her own health care. The movement has to a large extent sprung from women's insistence on their health needs and rights. Among its most dramatic results has been the re-examination and radical adjustment in the options offered for treatment of breast cancer. Women have demanded—with positive results—research on heart disease that covers women, not exclusively men as in the past. One of the most commonly used and dramatically effective treatments for ovarian cancer today is taxol, a medicine derived from the yew tree. Taxol was investigated and found effective by pharmaceutical company researchers with the support of the Natural Products Program of the National Institute of Cancer Research—an unconventional approach backed by a highly conventional government bureau.

Traditional and nontraditional physicians alike are learning that women want to hear more than just "the doctor's orders." They want to know if there are other possible treatments or approaches, and why the doctor is recommending one over the other. Women are beginning to ask whether the generally accepted treatment for a particular condition is always the most appropriate or if individual differences may call for variations. In the area of traditional hormone replacement, for example, there has recently been greater acceptance of the principle that "standard" doses and hormone replacement schedules work only for the small minority of women who fit a "standard" profile; the larger number of women need a tailor-made plan. As for health care in general, a recent survey showed that more and more medical doctors are now frequently prescribing what used to be considered fringe treatments: relaxation therapy (often for people with heart disease), biofeedback (for headaches and high blood pressure), self-help or support groups, and lifestyle modifications. The same survey showed that some 55 percent of alternative therapies were covered by health insurance, a surprising figure given the traditionally conservative attitude of insurance companies toward new, untried, or nonestablishment treatments.

Many leading nontraditional practitioners, at the same time, are becoming more willing to consider conventional therapies for women who are not likely to benefit from alternative or "natural" medicines. Women's menopause centers are being established across the country, and in most of them will be found accredited gynecologists and endocrinologists working together with naturopathic physicians, massage therapists, and other nonconventional practitioners such as herbalists. Nonconventional therapies may provide the best solution for women whose chief concerns are hot flashes or vaginal dryness, while hormone replacement is the only therapy proved effective in preventing or reducing the damage caused by osteoporosis.

In the case of something as complex as the functioning of reproductive hormones and the body's response to the major life changes of menstruation, childbearing, and menopause, alternative medicine is particularly relevant. For example, HRT may not be an option for women who have had breast or uterine cancer, uterine fibroids, liver disease, or blood-clotting problems, so natural remedies may be their first choice rather than a conventional treatment. Some women might not feel it is worth the potential complications and side effects to take hormones just for the milder symptoms of menopause such as occasional insomnia or vaginal dryness—which often can be completely relieved without estrogen. But many women have such severe symptoms and/or high risk for heart disease or osteoporosis or both, that the case for HRT is compelling.

But what is most significant for most women is just knowing there are options, that there is freedom of choice and that women themselves at least have a considerable degree of control over their health, present and future. Exploring alternatives has had another remarkable result: It has revealed evidence that women—and men—can make changes in their life habits that alone will improve their health, regardless of whether they choose a traditional or alternative approach as their primary therapy.

Q: What is "alternative" medicine?
A: In 1996, the National Library of Medicine issued its new definition of alternative medicine as "a group of nonorthodox therapeutic procedures that do not follow conventional biomedical explanations." This is an interesting upgrading from the library's previous definition, which was "nonorthodox therapeutic systems which have no satisfactory scientific explanation for their ef-

fectiveness." Another simpler and more common definition is "medical interventions that are not taught at United States medical schools or not available at United States hospitals." That definition may have to change, too, as more and more medical schools are beginning to look into alternative medicine in their research programs and to incorporate some of the basic alternative medicine principles (the holistic approach or "treating the whole person," for example) into their teaching programs.

Q: **What kind of treatments are included in alternative medicine?**
A: The list varies, according to the source. In 1993, a study of "unconventional" approaches reported in the *New England Journal of Medicine* included sixteen therapies in its definition: relaxation techniques, chiropractic, massage, therapeutic imagery, spiritual healing, commercial weight-loss programs, "lifestyle" diets such as macrobiotics, herbal medicine, megavitamin therapy, energy healing, biofeedback, hypnosis, homeopathy, acupuncture, folk remedies, and self-help groups. Others include new age healing, faith healing, music therapy, and "lifestyle modification."

Q: **Which of the unconventional approaches are used for estrogen deficiency or menopausal symptoms?**
A: They include approaches from almost every area of unconventional therapy: vitamins and

minerals, homeopathy, "natural" hormones, herbal medicine, dietary changes, massage, and acupuncture. In addition, for women who cannot take estrogen because of various risk factors (for example, women who have had breast cancer), conventional medical practitioners may prescribe progestin, megestol acetate, or clonidine. Calcitonin, alendronate, and calcium are known to inhibit bone breakdown and are used to prevent or treat osteoporosis. Some of the severe symptoms of menopause—insomnia, nervousness, hot flashes—may be relieved by mild sedatives, such as small doses of phenobarbitol and ergotamine. Rest, exercise, and good diet are considered an essential component of most alternative medicine approaches to menopause. Talking to other women in a support group can be quite helpful.

Alternative practitioners often emphasize the importance of mental attitude in the relief of menopausal symptoms. Without suggesting that your discomfort is "all in your mind," nevertheless they suggest that women who see menopause as a natural part of life tend to do better than those who view it negatively, as the end of youth and sexuality and true womanhood. Alternative practitioners also point out the importance of remembering, when making a decision about which form of therapy to use, that the decision does not have to be "forever." You can try one approach and if it does not work, switch to another. But they add that most natural remedies require a little more time than hormone replacement does, so you should not give up on it too quickly.

Q: Are any natural remedies considered exact substitutes for HRT?
A: Opinions differ. The reason a woman is seeking treatment in the first place—whether conventional or alternative—is the most significant factor in the answer. Natural approaches are more likely to work for more women in simply relieving hot flashes than for preventing hip fractures. For example, one of the most effective and simplest remedies for hot flashes is keeping your environment cool. Recent studies have shown that hot flashes occur six times as often when the temperature is about 88 or 89 degrees than when it is 67 or 68. In particular, most people keep their bedroom temperatures far too high at night; it has been shown that "night sweats" can be relieved or avoided entirely by using fewer or more "breathable" night clothes and bed covers and by lowering the room temperature at night.

One of the reasons menopausal women most often seek treatment is vaginal dryness, which is uncomfortable and can make intercourse painful, with all the attendant emotional and interpersonal problems this can entail. It is also one of the easiest to manage without HRT. Replens vaginal lotion is an over-the-counter remedy widely recommended by alternative practitioners, and there are a variety of vaginal lubricants that can be used before intercourse that can make you comfortable. If none of these work sufficiently well (which is rarely the case), your doctor can prescribe a topical estrogen cream. Some of the estrogen will be absorbed into your system but it will be a smaller amount compared to what you would take in standard HRT regimens.

Many natural remedies are not suggested as alternatives or adequate substitutes for hormones but as helpful adjuncts to hormone treatment, perhaps as a way of allowing a lower dose of hormones, or for women who are not at high risk for any of the principal postmenopausal health problems. For example: giving up cigarettes improves the circulation, reduces breathing problems, and increases stamina so that you can get more exercise, which is also healthful. But not even the most ardent proponent of natural remedies or the most fervent opponent of hormone replacement would claim that not smoking—by itself or even combined with other good health habits—is adequate preventive medicine for the woman with a decided family history of heart disease and a high cholesterol level that is not appropriately lowered by the correct diet.

Q: I have a friend who has been taking natural progesterone instead of estrogen and she swears by it. Is it as good as estrogen for menopause?

A: There is a school of thought, with proponents in both conventional and alternative camps, that argues in favor of progesterone—not estrogen—deficiency, as the real culprit in postmenopausal problems. Of course, progestin is added to estrogen in conventional HRT treatment, but some practitioners say it is not enough and others believe it should be given by itself, without estrogen and its potential problems. Natural progesterones are available over the counter and are often recommended by alternative practitioners. They may be taken in pill form or applied to the skin as a jelly or cream. Progesterone is believed to be effective not only against menopausal symptoms but in restoring bone. Because all hormones can be potent substances, alternative practitioners warn against self-prescribing and recommend getting expert advice—from a medical or alternative practitioner—before heading for the health food store.

Q: What vitamins and minerals are recommended?
A: Vitamins B_3, B_6, E, and C are the most common. Vitamin E is reported to stop hot flashes for many women. Folic acid, biotin, iodine, copper, selenium, and boron are said to increase calcium uptake and improve bone health. Vitamin A is suggested for healthy skin, eyes, and gums. A mineral extract called microcrystalline hydroxyapatite concentrate (MCHC) is used to help the body process calcium. Calcium supplements are recommended by various types of practitioners.

Q: Which herbal remedies are supposed to counteract estrogen deficiency?
A: Herbal medicine is an ancient art used for centuries in China. The most popular of the traditional Chinese herbs is dong quai (also known as

Angelic sinensis or just angelica). It is said to relieve hot flashes and calm menopausal anxiety. Dong quai is also rich in minerals such as magnesium and trace elements including cobalt. Another popular remedy is ginseng, a mainstay of Chinese herbal medicine, believed to function by restoring balance in body chemistry: in menopause it is recommended for rebalancing estrogen and progesterone. A variety of other herbs and their claimed effects include sage, which contains magnesium, calcium, and zinc, given a tablespoon at a time several times a day to ease night sweats and night flushes and to calm anxiety and relieve depression; motherwort, to ease hot flashes and relieve insomnia; Chasetree or Monks Pepper, believed to stimulate progesterone synthesis, relieve hot flashes, clear up hormone-associated skin problems, and regulate water retention. Among other popular remedies are sarsaparilla and licorice root. But herbalists caution that licorice can elevate blood pressure in people with hypertension. Wild yams or Mexican yams are recommended because they contain progesteronelike substances, and there is a widespread belief that progesterone is an even more significant key to menopausal good health than is estrogen. But wild yam sometimes causes intestinal distress.

Plants and herbs that are widely and strongly recommended for estrogen deficiency are those that contain phytoestrogens, the plant substance that is similar to human estrogen although not exactly the same. Tofu, made from soybeans, is the most widely used and abundant source of phytoestrogens, with soya bean milk also recommended. Other relatively common plants or vegetables that contain phytoestrogens include linseed, red clover, rhubarb, celery, and fennel.

Not so incidentally, it has recently been discovered by British researchers that tofu, in addition to plant estrogen, also contains isoflavenoids, the substances that are believed to block estrogen from contributing to the development of breast cancer. Isoflavenoids are the principal active ingredient in the widely used anticancer drug called tamoxifen.

Q: What is homeopathy?
A: It is a nonconventional treatment approach that uses very weak or diluted solutions of the substances that mimic the symptoms of a particular illness. Many scientists agree that in most cases the solutions have to be so diluted (to avoid actually producing symptoms) that they cannot have any effect at all. In any case, it is rarely used for estrogen deficiency.

Q: I've heard that evening primrose oil, which is often recommended to relieve premenstrual syndrome, is also helpful in menopause. What does it do?
A: Evening primrose oil and starflower oil, given along with minerals such as zinc and magnesium, are said to relieve the fatigue, tension, and depression that often accompany menopause. Evening primrose oil is one of the natural rem-

edies most likely to be suggested by conventional doctors for PMS (premenstrual syndrome) and for those specific symptoms of menopause (although not as a substitute for hormone replacement).

Q: Besides specific foods that contain plant estrogens, are there any other dietary changes that can counteract estrogen deficiency?
A: Not specifically, except perhaps in regard to hot flashes. Spicy foods, alcohol, and chocolate appear to worsen or trigger hot flashes, and many women have found relief by avoiding them. Dietary changes that are recommended for general health improvement that may offset some menopausal symptoms or stave off certain health risks of estrogen deficiency include eating more fresh and organic fruits and vegetables, and less dairy products and meat; eating more oily fish rich in omega-3 polyunsaturated fatty acids to improve cardiovascular health; drinking lots of water (one recommendation is a liter per 100 pounds of weight daily) to help the body rid itself of impurities and to reduce cravings for caffeine, which is deleterious to bones.

Q: What is tai chi chuan?
A: It is an ancient Chinese art that emphasizes balance and harmonious, flowing movement. It is considered potentially very helpful in protecting bones because it includes weight-bearing exercise and may help prevent falls and fractures because it improves balance and leg strength.

Q: What is acupuncture used for?
A: It is most often suggested for relieving depression and also for cramps during menstrual periods in early menopause or among those still having periods because of HRT.

Q: What lifestyle modifications are recommended by alternative practitioners?
A: They are very similar to those now being recommended by a great many mainstream practitioners. None is considered an alternative to estrogen, but singly and together they are believed to be helpful, even essential, in counteracting many of the symptoms and risks that come with estrogen deficiency. They include smoking cessation, which improves cardiovascular and pulmonary health and helps bones stay stronger; avoidance of caffeine, a calcium-depleter; reduction of both protein (which encourages bone loss) and fat (which raises the risk of heart disease and perhaps breast cancer); lower consumption of alcohol, which among other deleterious effects appears to increase cancer risk (50 percent higher among women who drink two to three drinks or more daily); reduction of stress (which makes symptoms worse) with massage, meditation, and bodywork.

Many women are surprised or even shocked when they are prompted by menopause to take a look at their eating, sleeping, and exercising patterns, and regardless of whether they choose traditional or nontraditional treatment for specific symptoms, begin to take better care of them-

selves in general, and to feel better than they did
even before menopause began. Taking a good
look at yourself, taking charge of your own
health, and making informed choices are excellent morale-boosters that add to your feeling of
well-being over and above the improvement resulting directly from changes in lifestyle.

Q: What kind of people tend to prefer alternative
medicine?

A: In 1990, a survey of 1,539 American adults
(reported in the *New England Journal of Medicine*)
revealed that unconventional therapies were
used most often by people between the ages of
twenty-five and forty-nine, those with some college education, and those with annual incomes
greater than $35,000. Among other interesting
findings of the survey was that some 10 percent
of all Americans got health care service in the
preceding year from an unconventional practitioner (chiropractor, herbal healer, or massage
therapist). About 25 percent more used some sort
of unconventional therapy on a self-prescribed
basis, without going to a practitioner. These therapies included large doses of vitamins, participation in self-help groups, or lifestyle changes.
Alternative therapy was most often sought for
back problems, anxiety, headaches, chronic pain,
and cancer.

Seven of ten people who used unconventional
therapy or saw an alternative medicine practitioner did not tell their regular medical doctor
about it. But that depended on the condition for

which they sought treatment. Only 4 percent visited an unconventional practitioner for treatment of arthritis, back pain, digestive problems or depression without also seeing a physician. Nobody who had cancer, diabetes, lung disease, skin disease, high blood pressure, urinary problems, or dental problems saw an unconventional therapist without also seeing a traditional practitioner.

The survey did not answer the question of how much of the alternative therapy was in fact recommended by a mainstream medical practitioner.

Among women likely to seek alternatives are those who have tried HRT and suffered side effects unpleasant or intolerable enough to make them quit. Some 80 percent of those for whom HRT has been prescribed drop out for one reason or another.

This study was the largest ever undertaken to analyze the use and cost of alternative medicine in this country. According to the report, Americans spent $13.7 billion for alternative medical care in 1990. Of this amount, most of it ($10.3 billion) came out of people's own pockets. During the same year Americans spent $12.8 billion out-of-pocket for hospital bills, while about $250 billion was paid for by insurance.

Q: **When alternative practitioners give you estrogen or other hormones, are they the same kind as regular physicians prescribe?**

A: They may be, although often they are so-called "natural hormones." These are made from plants and are similar to—but not identical to—the hormones produced by a woman's own glands and are known as "phytoestrogens." The most notable sources are tofu and other soybean-based products such as soya milk. "Natural" hormones also may be synthesized in a laboratory and are identical to human hormones—as are the various hormones used in standard HRT.

Q: Are natural hormones more effective or safer than the standard ones?
A: Nobody really knows the answer—regarding either effectiveness or safety. The research just has not been done yet or is still underway and the results not yet in. It has been suggested that plant hormones might be safe for women who have had breast cancer and should not take "real" estrogen, because the plant hormones are not the same and therefore would not have the same cancer-stimulating effect. But since they are different—and have not been extensively studied in controlled scientific trials—there is no currently available way of predicting whether they would behave differently or the same in any particular situation. Others claim that "natural" hormones are safer because they are not as strong or concentrated as those given in traditional HRT. Again, there is no research to support the claim.

As for effectiveness, the most compelling argument in favor of alternatives—specifically phytoestrogen—comes from comparisons of menopause in Japanese and American women. Tofu, which contains high concentrations of phytoestrogens, is a principal staple in the Japanese diet, and Japanese women have ten to forty times the level of phytoestrogens in their bloodstream than American women. They also report having menopausal hot flashes only one-sixth as often as American women. It is often noted as significant that there is no specific Japanese term for "hot flash."

Q: If tofu contains a kind of estrogen that could counteract menopausal symptoms, how much would I have to eat for it to do any good?

A: That is another open question. A little tofu mixed with stir-fried vegetables every few weeks or even every week—which is about the maximum most American women are likely to get normally—definitely cannot be expected to make much impact. Japanese women, who do not complain about menopausal symptoms as much as Western women, eat tofu just about every day, and in appreciable amounts. Researcher Margo Woods of Tufts University is conducting a study of one hundred women who eat a specially prepared soy candy bar every day for three months. The candy contains enough tofu to cover half a dinner plate—a sizeable enough amount to have a measurable effect if tofu does indeed reduce hot flashes. The results are not in.

Q: Do vitamins and minerals work against the symptoms of menopause?

A: Vitamin D and calcium are both thought to cut the long-term risks of osteoporosis due to estrogen deficiency. Some evidence suggests that vitamin E helps protect against heart disease and may relieve hot flashes. It has also been claimed—but not clearly demonstrated by research studies—that zinc chelate supplements can stimulate hormone production by the adrenal glands after it has declined in the ovaries.

Q: If I decide to try natural remedies instead of HRT, is there any way to tell if it's working as well as HRT would have?
A: There is probably no way to make a direct point-for-point comparison, since there is no way of telling exactly how HRT would have worked for you. Obviously, you will be able to tell whether any treatment is giving you relief from the symptoms that prompted you to seek help in the first place. You can find out if it is affecting your heart and bone health by having regular lipid profiles and bone density tests.

Q: Do natural remedies and treatments work equally well in protecting against heart disease and bone loss?
A: No. The natural approach that entails improved health habits such as exercise and better nutrition, not smoking, and avoiding excessive alcohol and caffeine consumption, can provide considerable protection against cardiovascular disease. These actions and calcium supplementation may be helpful in keeping bones healthy

but are probably inadequate for the one woman in three who is at high risk for osteoporosis.

Q: **Do menopause centers all offer choices among both traditional and alternative treatments?**
A: No, although many do. Others may focus exclusively on HRT, some on alternative therapies only (although these are less common) and some serve only as screening centers with referral to physicians or medical centers. Their quality also varies widely. You need to be on guard, for example, against unnecessary testing (bone densitometry, for example, if you have absolutely no risk factors for osteoporosis). Ask questions: Does the center have a multidisciplinary staff that includes at the very least a gynecologist and/or endocrinologist, an alternative practitioner, and a mental health specialist (psychiatrist, clinical social worker, or psychotherapist)? Will you have the option of choosing a woman for your primary caregiver? Does the center or the women's practice have an educational component? (Some centers sponsor open meetings where staff members talk about health issues of interest to women or educational sessions targeted specifically at menopause.) You may also find your needs may be met by a general women's health practice rather than a specialized menopause center.

Q: **My only really troublesome problem with menopause is depression, and I don't want to take**

hormones just for that. What about an antide-pressant?

A: Some doctors are quick to prescribe antide-pressants, especially the newer ones (such as Prozac) that have fewer side effects and are less physically addictive than earlier medications. But many doctors and most alternative practitioners oppose this practice. The sometimes tragic outcome of overeager prescribing of Valium and similar medicines when they were first introduced—which resulted in large numbers of women becoming seriously addicted and others of having their tendencies towards alcoholism complicated or exacerbated—have made many doctors wary. Others do not prescribe antide-pressants because they are convinced that the depression of menopause is hormonally based and therefore should be relieved by whatever treatment attacks the deficiency problem. Alternative practitioners in particular usually try to search for natural mood-altering therapies (such as nutrition, exercise, stress reduction) to combat depression and other emotional imbalances.

Q: **I've followed natural health recommendations for many years, eating little fat, using organic products whenever possible, getting plenty of exercise, and avoiding meats, tobacco, alcohol, and caffeine, but now I'm suffering from really severe menopausal symptoms and am at high risk for osteoporosis. Will natural remedies work for me?**

A: They might. Some alternative medicine specialists firmly believe that *nobody* should take HRT, certainly not for the ten or twenty years that appear necessary for adequate protection against osteoporosis. But many naturopaths or other alternative practitioners would suggest that you may be one of the people for whom they would certainly recommend HRT. Few such practitioners claim that natural remedies are the solution for every health problem. You should definitely consult with a medical doctor—perhaps an endocrinologist or other specialist in menopause—and an alternative practitioner. A bone-density study might be considered, to find out whether osteoporosis is already affecting you.

Q: **I'm not so sure that my main symptoms, which are insomnia, irritability, dizziness, and particularly chronic fatigue, are really due to menopause; is there any way to find out and any way to get relief besides hormones?**

A: Those symptoms are certainly common in menopause and may—or may not—be related to estrogen deficiency. You could ask your doctor to check your estrogen levels. You could also talk to your doctor or an alternative practitioner or even do a self-assessment to find out what stresses in your life may be causing or enhancing these symptoms. Menopause happens at a time when many other disturbing changes may be taking place: imminent retirement (which is a stressful change even if you are looking forward to it); financial insecurity because of the overall economy or declining personal productivity; extra pressure at work as you rise to higher levels of responsibility; caring for elderly or ill parents; dealing with children who are entering high-tension years (college, marriage, or first pregnancy); concerns triggered by societal attitudes toward older people; fear of aging; or loss of attractiveness to your sexual partner.

Many of these stresses can be addressed and relieved by various nonmedical actions. Talking with a counselor or joining a support group is a good first step. Examining and correcting bad eating, sleeping, and exercise patterns and getting rid of unhealthy habits such as smoking and excessive drinking can result in major improvement. Most important is to give yourself permission to be good to yourself: Take fifteen minutes (better still, a half hour) a day to be absolutely private and quiet to read, relax in a tub, nap, walk in the park, or just meditate. Exercise—the more strenuous the better, with your doctor's approval—can be an amazing stress-reducer. Brisk walking is good, but often the companionship and fun of group exercise can enhance the effect of the physical exertion. Doubles tennis or doubles platform tennis (one of the few sports other than skiing that you can still do outdoors in the winter) can be played at any age or any level of skill or physical capacity if you find suitable companions. (Meanwhile, the exercise is helping you protect your bones.)

Q: I've heard about something called "stress management" for dealing with fatigue, depression,

and irritability. What is it and where do you get it?

A: Generally speaking, stress management consists of several basic techniques or approaches for relieving emotional and physical pressure. Some people consider "management" a misnomer that unfortunately suggests a busy executive organizing and dealing with a welter of details and problems. Stress "reduction" might be a more accurate term, since the goal is to help you eliminate some of the stresses in your life and relieve your response to those that are unavoidable. The elimination process may begin simply with identifying what the stressors are and removing or minimizing them; for example, learning how better to delegate some of the responsibilities of your job, asking your family to take a greater share in your household workload, giving up some optional volunteer work, learning how to say "no" to unreasonable requests from family or friends. Relieving your stress responses may involve one or more of these basic techniques.

- Biofeedback training: This entails the use of a machine that measures your heart rate, blood pressure, and skin temperature. A biofeedback trainer guides you through a relaxation exercise (which may include counting slowly backward, imagining a pleasant scene, meditating and using a mantra or repeated silent chanting of a word or syllable, or relaxing all your muscles one by one, starting with your forehead and working very slowly down to your toes). As you practice the exercise, the machine signals you that the telltale measurements are successfully being reduced or relaxed. This "feedback" tends to encourage and permanently imprint the successful relaxation technique, so that you can practice it at home without the machine.

- Breathing exercises: Used alone or with biofeedback, this technique involves first focusing on your breathing and becoming aware of the air moving in and out of one or both nostrils, then taking slow, deep breaths so that you have a relaxed, controlled breathing rhythm.

- Positive imagery: This involves trying to recall the sight, sound, smell, and emotions you experienced during an intensely pleasant time in your life, or of imagining such an experience. Another form of positive imagery involves visualizing some imaginary person or thing (for example, a crowd of friendly aliens or elves) working inside you to conquer your symptoms.

One approach to stress management is simply short-term psychotherapy with a practitioner who has a special interest in this area, short-term meaning perhaps ten or twelve therapy sessions.

Your primary health care giver or psychotherapist may be able to refer you to an appropriate source of stress management.

Q: **My older sister had breast cancer and I've heard that I shouldn't take hormones but I'm worried about osteoporosis and afraid that alternative therapy won't be sufficient. What should I do?**

A: Talk to your doctor and perhaps to an alternative practitioner about it. Some doctors do not think that such a family history is enough to rule out HRT; some do not even think that if you had breast cancer yourself and were successfully treated means you absolutely should avoid hormone replacement. A nationally known expert in women's health, Dr. Lila Wallis of Cornell University Medical College, had this to say in the *Journal of the American Medical Women's Association*:

> . . . not every history of breast cancer in a mother or sister has the same weight. When the patient is severely symptomatic or profoundly vulnerable to osteoporosis, I would assiduously search, along with the patient, for a reason *not* to consider such first-degree family history an absolute contraindication. I would entertain the possibility of linkages among such visible traits as height, body structure, skin and hair coloring with the genetic predisposition to various cancers. I would ask the patient: "Do you resemble your mother (or sister) in appearance or temperament? Or are you more like the paternal

side of the family?'' Perhaps in the future, such linkages will be provable by epidemiological research, and if the patient's appearance is sufficiently different from that of her affected relative, we could remove that contraindication in her case.

Another important point is the reason for your worries about osteoporosis. If the condition is widespread among your closest female relatives, or if you already have symptoms or have had a bone density examination that reveals a problem, that is one thing. If you are just worried on the general grounds that osteoporosis is a danger for women after a certain age, that is an entirely different matter. If the latter, you certainly could make a case for alternative medicine. What you need most is enough information and knowledgeable advice to allow you to make a decision well grounded in fact and in an understanding of all your possible options.

NINE

༺✦༻

Your Choice: How to Find the Right Doctor

CASE STUDY

Edna, a 55-year-old grandmother, had gone to the same family physician for nearly ten years. Most of her visits involved minor ailments, so the time that she spent with her doctor was usually brief. But when Edna began to experience the first symptoms of menopause—insomnia, poor concentration, and what she called "the blahs"—she started seeing her physician more frequently and came to realize that he was not as caring and compassionate as she had thought.

"He didn't seem particularly concerned with the various problems I was having at the onset of menopause, and often acted as if they were all in my head. When I asked questions about my treatment, his answers were never very specific. He just didn't make me feel very good at all."

Edna continued to visit her doctor for a couple of months but she was still dissatisfied. Her daughter, a patient of mine, realized how miserable Edna was and encouraged her to find a more compassionate practitioner. She also felt that her mother might be more comfortable with a female doctor.

I gave Edna the name of a female OB/GYN who specialized in menopause management. She made an appointment for an initial visit. "My new physician was much friendlier, and showed much more concern for what I was going through," Edna said. "She took a lot of notes, asked questions, and took the time to discuss my options at length. She told me I had a lot of treatment alternatives, and gave me plenty of time to make up my mind. The difference was like night and day.

"I now tell my friends that they're not married to their doctors, and if they don't like the treatment they're receiving, they should look for another physician. It can make a big difference."

Your doctor will be your guide throughout menopause. But he is only one-half of the partnership. By combining your doctor's medical expertise with your own knowledge of what is right for you, you can make informed decisions about your health. The result is often a change of life unattended by fear or discomfort.

Some women choose to stay with their family physician or gynecologist. Others feel more comfortable consulting now and then with an endocrinologist or other specialist. The key is to find a skilled practioner with whom you feel comfortable, who listens to and understands your concerns, who educates you about what is happening inside your body, and provides detailed and easy to understand information about all your treatment options.

In this chapter, you will learn how to intelligently go about finding the right physician for you, what questions to ask, and how to get the most from your doctor-patient relationship. But remember, even the most talented and skilled doctor depends on your active participation in order to provide the best care for you.

Q: **I've been seeing the same gynecologist for nearly twenty years. I'm premenopausal, and wondering if I should stay with him for care during my change of life. What are my options when it comes to physicians?**

A: When it comes to the management of menopause, you have three options: a general practice family physician, a gynecologist, or a hormone specialist such as an endocrinologist.

Of the three, most women opt to stay with their gynecologist when menopause occurs. Because they are specialists in the female reproductive system, most gynecologists are quite up to date on the latest menopause treatments, including the advantages and potential problems of HRT. More importantly, if you have been going to the same doctor for twenty years, he obviously is well aware of your ongoing medical history and thus able to make informed decisions on what management strategies would be best for you.

A family physician may also be knowledgeable when it comes to the management of menopause, but generally speaking, most are not. Their practices tend to cover a wider area of medical problems, and while many family physicians provide very good gynecological care, they may be unaware of the very latest developments in menopause treatment.

An endocrinologist is most often consulted when a patient needs a specific test, or experiences problems caused by menopause-related hormone disturbances. Care from such specialists tends to be more costly than that of a family practitioner or gynecologist, and it makes little sense to see one if you do not have to. In most cases, consultation with an endocrinologist will come at the referral of your primary care physician.

Q: Are there different kinds of endocrinologists? Does it matter which one I go to? Do I need a specialist at all?
A: There are two kinds of endocrine system specialists. Medical endocrinologists are usually doctors who qualify in internal medicine and then take additional training to specialize in the endocrine system. Reproductive endocrinologists are gynecologists who take additional training in the female endocrine system and infertility. You may get excellent treatment from either one—but you would be wise to find out exactly what their main concerns are—whether the medical endocrinologist has experience in managing women's

hormonal health, or whether the reproductive endocrinologist is focused on menopause and HRT or is mostly interested in infertility. Almost every doctor has learned something about female hormones during their medical training, and even your family doctor may have far more experience with women's health problems than a newly certified specialist. Sensitivity to women's health issues is sometimes more important than training. But if you have hormonal problems or menopausal symptoms that really concern you, or if you want the best possible advice about the risks and benefits of hormone treatment, then you should learn as much as you can about the expert you intend to consult.

Q: Should I see a male or female gynecologist for the management of my menopause symptoms? Does it really make a difference in quality of care?
A: Whether to choose a male or female gynecologist to help you through menopause is a decision only you can make. Some women feel quite comfortable with their male doctors and see no reason to switch, while others believe that a female physician would be more sympathetic to the needs and emotions of a female patient on the verge of menopause.

This issue has been the subject of debate for decades. Some people—including many physicians—feel that men have certain disadvantages as gynecologists because they have no frame of reference for what a woman experiences physically and emotionally over the course of her life. Male doctors, say detractors, tend to ignore or downplay many of the physical symptoms related to menopause—physical symptoms for which a female doctor would show greater concern. Others argue that a physician is a physician regardless of gender, and that a properly trained male doctor is as concerned and sympathetic toward his patients as a female physician.

Some women are uncomfortable being examined by or talking to male physicians, and benefit more from seeing female doctors. A doctor-patient relationship that is hindered by anxiety or embarrassment is counterproductive.

Get some input from a female friend or family member. Is her doctor male or female? Does she feel comfortable with her physician? Does her doctor listen to her complaints, enlist her input, and actively involve her in treatment? All of these are important issues that must be taken into consideration when choosing a physician— especially one who will be guiding you through menopause.

Q: **My husband and I just moved into town, and we're still getting settled. I am approaching menopause and anxious to talk to a doctor about it. How should I go about finding a physician who's right for me?**

A: There are many ways to find a doctor. The telephone book is one way to go about it, but I would not recommend it. Most of the time all you get is a simple listing that tells you little about a doctor's qualifications or expertise. A more effective option would be to contact your local medical association or hospital and ask for a listing of gynecologists in your area. Many referral organizations will also fill you in on a doctor's special qualifications or areas of expertise, whether he is board certified (which is a definite plus), and whether he has had any malpractice suits filed against him.

If your local medical association or hospital cannot help you, consult a female friend or co-worker, especially one who is under a doctor's care for the management of menopause. Is she happy with her doctor and the treatment she is receiving? Would she recommend her physician to others? What does she like most about her doctor? What does she like least? Is her doctor seeing new patients? Many times word of mouth is a tremendous source of valuable information.

Q: Once I've made a short list of potential doctors, what should I do?

A: Make an appointment to meet with each of them, then ask lots of questions. It is very important that you feel comfortable with the physician you choose because you will be spending a lot of time together discussing your health concerns and you will probably be touching on many personal issues over the course of your relationship.

Things to look for in your new physician include the following.

- A willingness to meet with you before accepting you as a patient. Most doctors do not like being "shopped," but sometimes a sensitive physician will understand your motives.

- Good communication skills that include active listening and a friendly manner.

- A willingness to answer simple questions over the telephone.

- A keen interest in preventive medicine and wellness education. A good doctor-patient relationship should involve much more than mere treatment when you are ill—it should also involve prevention.

- A willingness to explain medical recommendations to you in plain English, and to discuss medical alternatives if necessary.

- A courteous, friendly office staff.

Q: What kinds of questions should I ask a prospective doctor during our initial meeting? I want to make sure I cover all the bases.

A: Your initial meeting should be more of a friendly chat than a formal interview, but there are several specific questions that you should ask. Just to be on the safe side, you might want to write them down so you do not forget them.

The most important questions include the following.

- What are the doctor's credentials? Is she board-certified?

- How many patients does the doctor schedule in an hour? A very heavy load means less time for you.

- How far in advance must you schedule an appointment for a checkup? If she is unavailable for the next six months, you might want to find a doctor who is a little more accessible.

- How difficult is it to get a same-day appointment when you are really sick?

- Does she schedule time for emergency visits?

- Does she offer after-hour or weekend appointments? Is someone on call during nonbusiness hours?

- What is her attitude and approach toward illness prevention? Does she provide helpful literature?

- Does her practice include nurse practitioners or physician assistants?

- What is her attitude and approach regarding the management of menopause?

- Does she treat a lot of patients with this condition?

- How does she feel about HRT and related management techniques? Some doctors actively disapprove of HRT, while others prefer to evaluate it on a case by case basis. It may be helpful to talk to both kinds of doctors.

Q: **My doctor has a lot of certificates on his wall, but it's hard to tell what they really mean. How can I verify my doctor's medical credentials?**
A: It is always a good idea to verify your doctor's credentials if you have any doubt at all. The vast majority of physicians are well-trained, honest practitioners. A call to your state or local medical society should help you in confirming your doctor's credentials.

Q: **How can I tell if my doctor is board certified, and is that important?**
A: A doctor who is board certified has undergone additional training and passed an examination in a particular specialty. If your doctor says she is board certified, you can confirm it by calling the American Board of Medical Specialties (ABMS), located in Evanston, Illinois. It contains twenty-four member boards (including the American Board of Obstetrics and Gynecology) that govern certification in thirty-eight general specialties and seventy-four subspecialties. The toll-free number, available Monday through Friday between 9 a.m. and 6 p.m. EST, is 800-776-2378.

It is important to note that there are more than 120 self-designated specialty boards that are *not* recognized by the American Board of Medical Specialties. Some require extensive training, while others will sell certification for just a few dollars.

Board certification offers many advantages in addition to more medical training and expertise. In fact, a lot of hospitals will not allow admitting or surgical privileges to doctors who are not board-certified. And studies show that board-certified physicians are involved in far fewer medical lawsuits.

Q: I always get flustered when I visit my doctor and sometimes forget to bring up important issues I'd like to discuss. What can I do to make the time I have with my doctor more productive?

A: It is a common problem. Many women make a mental list of things they want to mention to their doctor, only to forget half of them once they are on the examining table. One of the easiest solutions to this problem is to write down the things you want to talk about with your doctor, and bring the list with you when you go. Most doctors appreciate this extra effort because it suggests that the patient is taking an active interest in her health and well-being. It is also a good idea to show some initiative when talking with your doctor. Physicians are busy people, and may forget to bring up a specific issue or assume it is not a problem if you do not mention it first.

A few more tips to help you get the most from your doctor visits follow.

- If you have them, bring all your medical records with you when visiting a doctor for the first time. This will give him a complete understanding of your medical history.

- Keep a health diary between visits, if appropriate, and write down significant changes in a specific condition or your health in general. This will help you remember what you want to discuss when you finally see your doctor.

- Always discuss your symptoms and problems in detail. Do not leave anything out because you are embarrassed or afraid. Silence only endangers your health.

- If you do not understand what your doctor is saying to you, ask him to speak in plain English. Repeat the request until you are certain that you understand everything.

- Ask your doctor if he has any literature on your problem. Having information in writing often makes it easier to understand.

- If your doctor writes you a prescription, ask him what it is for, how much you should take, and for how long you should take it, when and how you should take it (on a full or empty stomach?), and ask about any potential side effects. Double check this information with the pharmacist when you get the prescription filled.

- If your doctor wants to schedule you for

a test, ask what the procedure is for, what it entails, how much it costs, and whether there are any less costly or less invasive alternatives. You should also ask when the results will be ready, who will interpret them, and how you will be contacted.

Q: I hate to bother my doctor when it comes to minor health questions. Could you suggest some resources for general health and medical information?

A: Your local library is a good place to start. There are more health and medical books available now than ever before, and most libraries carry a sizable selection. In addition, you might want to check the Index Medicus, which provides a complete index of articles published in the major medical journals (which most libraries also carry). If your library has online computers ask your librarian about accessing MEDLINE (the online version of Index Medicus) through the Bethesda-based National Library of Medicine.

If you are looking to create a home medical library, you should consider the following.

- *The American Medical Association Encyclopedia of Medicine*
- *The Encyclopedia of Health Information Sources*
- *The Encyclopedia of Medical Organizations and Agencies*

- *The Mayo Clinic Family Health Book*
- *The Merck Manual of Diagnosis and Therapy*
- *The Oxford Textbook of Medicine*
- *The Wellness Encyclopedia*

People who own home computers have a special advantage because many excellent health and medical books are available on CD-ROM, and most are very reasonably priced. In addition to text, most medical CDs also offer graphics, and even short video clips.

If you have a computer but not a CD-ROM, do not despair. Most of the major online companies, such as Prodigy, Genie, and CompuServe, provide a number of excellent health forums. Some are general, while others are very specific; some are reviewed by physicians, while others are merely a place for like-minded individuals to meet and share information. But remember, people can say just about anything they want to on an open forum, which means there is a lot of misinformation floating around. Most online medical forums should be viewed only as a source of ideas, not authoritative medical information. Thoroughly research anything that you read.

Finally, for a list of all government agencies offering free health information, call the National Center for Health Information toll-free at 800-336-4797.

Q: A friend told me that there's a Patient Bill of Rights. Is this true? What is it?

A: The Patient Bill of Rights was conceived in 1992 by the American Hospital Association. It states, among other things, the following.

- You have the right to considerate and respectful care.

- You have the right to be well informed about your illness, possible treatments, and likely outcome, and to discuss this information with your doctor. You have the right to know the names and roles of the people treating you.

- You have the right to consent to or to refuse a treatment, as permitted by law, throughout your hospital stay. If you refuse a recommended treatment, you will receive other needed and available care.

- You have the right to privacy. The hospital, your doctor, and others caring for you will protect your privacy as much as possible.

- You have the right to expect that treatment records are confidential unless you have given permission to release information or reporting is required by law. When the hospital releases records to others, such as insurers, it emphasizes that the records are confidential.

- You have the right to review your medical

records and to have the information explained, except when restricted by law.

- You have the right to know about hospital rules that affect you and your treatment, and about charges and payment methods. You have the right to know about hospital resources, such as patient representatives or an ethics committee, that can help you resolve problems and questions about your hospital stay and care.

Q: My doctor is great when it comes to managing the symptoms of menopause, but he doesn't have a particularly friendly bedside manner. He tends to be gruff and rather stern, which bothers me a lot. What should I do?

A: The best thing you can do is tell your doctor exactly how you feel the next time you see him. You would be doing him a favor since he is probably unaware of how his personality affects his patients. If the idea of a confrontation intimidates you, talk with one of his nurses. If, after your talk, your doctor is not any friendlier, you have two options—tolerate his gruff demeanor, or find another doctor.

Q: I get the impression that my doctor does not view my menopause symptoms or other health complaints as seriously as I do. Any advice on how I can change this situation?

A: First, take a moment to reevaluate how concerned you appear during office visits. Doctors usually treat their patients based on how the patients treat themselves. If you come across as indifferent or lighthearted when discussing your health, your doctor will most likely assume the same attitude.

It is true that some doctors do not take the complaints of their female patients as seriously as they do those of their male patients, but that attitude is becoming increasingly rare as medical science continues to confirm the biological basis for the most common menopause problems. But if you feel that your doctor is being unprofessional, tell him point-blank about your concerns. And if you do not like his answers, find another doctor. Do not continue to see a physician with whom you feel uncomfortable.

Q: **I know what I expect from my doctor—respect, courtesy, and skilled medical care—but what does he expect from me as a patient? Is there anything I can do to make our relationship run even more smoothly?**

A: That is an excellent question, and one that all doctors will appreciate. When dealing with your doctor, you should always practice the Golden Rule—do unto him as you would have him do unto you. You expect respect and courtesy, and you should reciprocate in kind. Too often patients treat their physicians like hired help, which does not improve a doctor-patient relationship.

There are other things that doctors expect from their patients as well. For example, when making an appointment, explain your reason for wanting to see the doctor. The amount of time set aside for your visit is based on the information you provide. But many patients come in for one thing, then mention half a dozen other complaints while they are there. That eats up time the doctor has scheduled for other patients.

It also helps if you do a little homework regarding your medical condition. If you educate yourself about your condition, you are more likely to be aware of subtle changes that may be important to your care and recovery.

You should also do what your doctor tells you. His advice is based on expected results, which may not occur if you do not follow his instructions. If he gives you a prescription, for example, have it filled right away and take it as suggested. If he recommends a change in diet, then do it. Do not ignore your doctor's advice, or worse, try to self-medicate if he recommends a particular course of treatment.

Q: I really love my gynecologist. She's sensitive, compassionate, and very knowledgeable. But I can't say the same for some members of her office staff. Often they're belligerent and just plain rude. How should I handle this?

A: Inform your physician whenever a member of her office staff behaves less than professionally. The front office personnel are the first people a patient sees, and their actions reflect upon the entire practice—good or bad. It is likely that your doctor is unaware of her staff's poor behavior, and she will probably appreciate your comments. The next time any member of your doctor's staff is rude or obnoxious, let the person know that you do not appreciate their behavior, and notify the doctor immediately.

Q: **My gynecologist has strongly suggested that I consider ERT for my menopause symptoms, but I'm unsure if that's what I really need. Would it be appropriate for me to get a second opinion?**

A: Absolutely. A second opinion can be a valuable aid when making a serious medical decision, and ERT certainly qualifies. Your doctor should have no problem with this decision, and may even be able to suggest a handful of qualified doctors for you to contact. If he cannot or will not, call your local hospital or medical society for the names of area doctors who specialize in menopause management. If you keep hearing the same name over and over, that is a good recommendation for the best person to consult.

A second opinion may be sought for a variety of medical situations. The most common include the following.

- You are unsure if your doctor's diagnosis is correct.
- Your doctor says that there is nothing that can be done.
- You feel uncomfortable about recommended surgery.

- You have concern about your illness or your doctor's recommended treatment.

Before getting a second opinion, check with your insurance company to make sure that you are covered. Not all health plans reimburse clients for the cost of a second opinion.

Q: **The cost of medical care seems to get higher and higher every day. As I approach menopause, is there anything I can do to keep my medical expenses down?**

A: Most people think that the cost of medical care is set in stone, but that is not true. There are many things you can do to keep your costs to a minimum.

Most importantly, remain healthy. Staying out of the doctor's office is the best way to avoid high medical costs. Try using self-care for minor problems. Going to the doctor when it is unnecessary is an easy way to run up an astronomical bill. If you do end up visiting the doctor, ask how much you will be paying for a certain procedure or service. You would not buy a new television without knowing the price, and the same philosophy goes for your health care. Ask your doctor up front about the cost, and if it is expensive, ask him about less costly alternatives.

It might also help to negotiate with your doctor regarding price or terms. For example, some doctors offer discounts to patients who pay up front or file their own insurance claims. It cannot hurt to ask, and you might be pleasantly surprised. You should also keep a detailed medical journal containing a record of your doctor visits, lab tests, prescriptions, and related items. Ask for an itemized bill, and check it against your log to make sure that you are not paying for something you have not received. This is especially true if you have been in the hospital, where billing errors are rampant. If you have any questions, call immediately for an explanation.

Reduce your medical test costs by always questioning whether or not they are necessary. Sometimes doctors prescribe tests as standard procedure, or they are trying to protect themselves from a malpractice suit. These are *not* good reasons for undergoing a test, especially if you are paying for it. Remember: No test can be done without your consent. If you feel it is unnecessary, say so.

Finally, if your doctor gives you a prescription, ask if it is really needed. If so, ask about the availability of a less costly generic version, or better still, an over-the-counter equivalent. The difference in price can be significant.

Q: **I would like to try ERT for my menopause problems, but my doctor says he doesn't believe in it. Other than this disagreement, I really like him. How can I get him to consider my request?**

A: Have you asked your doctor why he is so adamantly against ERT? If not, you should. Communication is one of the strongest components of a good doctor-patient relationship, and it sounds as if you and your doctor are not communicating effectively.

Ask your doctor if he is against ERT in general, or if he thinks it is not appropriate for you. If the latter is true, you need to find out why. Is there something in your medical history that suggests ERT would be ineffective or dangerous? Or does he just want to try other alternative therapies first?

If your doctor simply dislikes ERT, but you feel it would be right for you, you might want to consider getting a second opinion to validate your claim. A doctor who dismisses his patient's comments and requests without a detailed explanation may not have his patient's best interests at heart.

Q: I'm a vegetarian who is interested in holistic remedies. I'm starting to suffer minor discomfort as a result of menopause, and would like to try some natural remedies before resorting to drugs or HRT. But my gynecologist scoffs at the idea. How can I find a holistic or naturopathic physician who will help me?

A: Most conventional doctors are at least willing to try a well-established natural remedy if a patient requests it, but many are still uncomfortable with any form of treatment outside the mainstream. This is unfortunate, because many women have reported a marked reduction in menopause symptoms after trying various natural remedies.

To find a doctor more in tune with your thinking, you may wish to contact the American Association of Naturopathic Physicians (P.O. Box 20386, Seattle, WA 98102; tel: 206-323-7610) or the American Holistic Medical Association (4101 Lake Boone Trail, #201, Raleigh, NC 27607; tel: 919-787-5146).

Q: **I'm using specific herbs and other natural remedies to help alleviate hot flashes and other symptoms of menopause, and they work well. But must I tell my doctor I'm doing this? I don't know how he would react.**

A: Yes, you definitely should tell your primary care physician that you are taking herbs and trying other alternative therapies—even if you think he will not like the idea. The reason is simple: Some natural remedies can have side effects or affect other body systems, so it is important that your doctor stay informed. Just because he does not approve does not mean that you should stop—especially if the remedy is working. But pay attention if he expresses specific concerns. Herbal therapy and other natural remedies are not for everyone.

Q: **I'm concerned about how menopause will affect my sexuality, but every time I mention it to my doctor, he blushes and changes the subject. Any advice?**

A: Most people believe that doctors know everything there is to know about the workings of the human body—including sex. But in truth, human sexuality, aside from related diseases, is either ignored completely or touched on only briefly in most medical schools. As a result, many doctors working today have only minimal knowledge of sex and libido. And that can be bad news for their patients.

It sounds like your doctor is a little embarrassed by the topic of sex, which could explain why he changes the subject and does not address your concerns. You could force the issue the next time you see him (which may or may not be effective) or you could consult another physician. A gynecologist who specializes in the management of menopause, for example, would almost certainly be able to answer your questions and help you approach menopause as a sexually happy and healthy woman. Another option is to consult a sex therapist with a strong background in geriatric sexuality.

Regardless of whom you consult, make sure that you talk to someone. Menopause can have a dramatic impact on a woman's sexuality and it is important that you and your partner be prepared.

Glossary

acupuncture: Chinese practice of inserting very thin needles into certain sites on the body to treat illnesses, to relieve stress or pain, or to induce anesthesia for surgery.

adrenal glands: endocrine glands located above each kidney that excrete hormones like epinephrine and cortisone.

amenorrhea: abnormal absence of menstruation that is a symptom of many diseases and conditions.

androstenedione: male sex hormone, weaker than testosterone; secreted by the testis, ovary, and adrenal cortex.

angioplasty: procedure to eliminate areas that have narrowed in blood vessels.

anorexia: loss of appetite for food. Anorexia nervosa is a mental disorder found predominantly in females beginning during adolescence. This disease is characterized by the refusal to eat, the fear of being obese despite marked weight loss, and interruption of the menstrual cycle. Hospitalization is often necessary to prevent starvation.

arteriosclerosis: disease characterized by the hardening and thickening of artery walls, resulting in decreased elasticity.

atherosclerosis: form of arteriosclerosis characterized by the hardening and thickening of artery walls and by fatty deposits on the inner walls.

biofeedback training: behavior modification technique in which an individual is given information, usually in auditory or visual mode, regarding his involuntary body functions, such as blood pressure, heart rate or skin temperature; this technique may help an individual gain voluntary control of those body functions. Used for stress management.

calcitonin: hormone secreted from the thyroid gland that helps to lower the level of calcium in blood plasma.

calcium: essential mineral found in bones and teeth. Also needed for the proper functioning of certain organs and muscles.

carpal tunnel syndrome: condition caused by the compression of a nerve that passes through the hand and wrist; it is characterized by loss of sensation and pain, and is caused by activities that require repetitive motion, such as typing.

climacteric: another term for menopause.

collagen: fibrous protein found in skin, bone, cartilage, and all other connective tissue.

congestive heart failure: heart failure resulting from weakened heart muscles that are unable to pump enough blood; characterized by breathlessness and abnormal retention of water and sodium.

coronary heart disease: damage of the heart muscle due to fatty plaque buildup in the coronary arteries resulting in an insufficient supply of oxygenated blood to the heart.

corticosteroid: any one of twenty-one steroids produced by the adrenal gland; used for hormonal replacement therapy.

depilatory: topical substance used to remove body hair.

dual energy x-ray absorptiometry (DEXA): procedure that uses very low levels of radiation to measure bone density.

endocrine system: network of glands that release hormones into the bloodstream that control growth, the digestive and reproductive systems, and other processes.

endocrinologist: doctor who specializes in the diagnosis and treatment of disorders of the endocrine glands.

endometrial hyperplasia: abnormal overgrowth of the mucous membrane lining the uterus.

endometrium: mucous membrane that lines the uterus which is shed during menstruation.

ergotamine: substance used to treat migraine headaches.

estradiol: very potent ovarian and placental estrogenic hormone that occurs naturally or can be synthetically produced, sometimes used to treat menopausal symptoms.

estriol: crystalline estrogenic hormone found in high concentrations in human pregnancy urine; a product (through oxidation) of estradiol and estrone.

estrogen: female sex hormone, responsible for development of female secondary sex characteristics. Produced in the endocrine gland, ovary, fatty tissue, placenta, and testis; can be produced synthetically.

estrogen receptors: regulatory protein on a cell surface, that binds estrogenic hormones.

estrone: estrogenic hormone that is found in high concentrations in male and human pregnancy urine, human plasma, palm kernel oil, and in some mammal urine; can be produced synthetically.

etidronate: compound that inhibits the resorption and deposition of certain minerals in bone. Used in bone scanning and to treat Paget's bone disease.

familial hyperlipidemia: hereditary disorder in which there is an excess of fat or lipids present in the blood.

fibrinogen: plasma protein produced in the liver which is converted to fibrin, a protein involved in blood clotting.

fibrocystic: presence of cysts and overgrowth of fibrous tissues.

follicle (ovarian): sac or tubular gland containing a developing egg in the ovary.

follicle-stimulating hormone (FSH): hormone produced by the pituitary gland which stimulates estrogen secretion and the growth of follicles in the ovary.

gland: cell or group of cells that process material from your bloodstream for further use in the body or for elimination.

gonadotropin: hormone that stimulates the gonads.

hormone replacement therapy: treatment that elevates lowered estrogen levels by providing replacement estrogen with a form of progesterone.

hot flashes: sudden, brief sensations of heat, often accompanied by sweating and chills; usually associated with menopause.

hypertension: high blood pressure.

hypothalamus: part of the brain above the pituitary gland. Controls many functions such as body temperature, sleep, appetite, etc.

hysterectomy: surgical procedure in which the entire uterus is removed.

incontinence: inability to control the bladder or bowels.

insomnia: inability to get adequate sleep, which can be occasional or a long-term condition.

in vitro fertilization: removal of an egg from the female and its fertilization in an artificial environment (like a test tube), and placement of fertilized egg back into the uterus of the same (or another) female.

kidney: one of a pair of organs that excrete waste products of metabolism.

libido: sexual drive or desire.

lipoprotein: lipid-protein complex which transports lipids (fats) in the blood.

low-density lipoprotein (LDL): class of lipid-protein complexes in the blood responsible for transporting cholesterol to the liver.

luteinizing hormone (LH): hormone produced by the pituitary that acts with FSH to stimulate ovulation, and androgen and progesterone secretion.

mammogram: X ray of the breast.

mantra: form of prayer.

menopause: period of time when menstruation ceases, usually occurring around age fifty.

menses: menstrual flow.

mestranol: synthetic estrogen used in oral contraceptives.

myocardial infarction: heart attack; degeneration of the heart muscle that results from inadequate blood supply to the area.

naturopathic physician: physician who uses a drugless system of therapy.

neurotransmitter: chemical that transmits nerve impulses across the synapse of two neurons.

norgestimate: hormone found in the corpus luteum, a glandular mass which forms after a follicle has ruptured.

oophorectomy: removal of one or both ovaries.

osteoporosis: condition that usually affects older women, characterized by a decrease in bone mass, increasing fragility and susceptibility to fractures.

ovary: female reproductive organ that produces eggs; typically found in pairs.

ovulation: production and discharge of eggs from the ovaries.

pancreas: large gland that secretes enzymes and the hormones insulin and glucagon.

Pap test: procedure in which cells are scraped from the cervix and examined under a microscope for any abnormalities.

perimenopausal: around the time of menopause.

phenobarbital: long-acting barbituate taken orally as a sedative, anticonvulsant, or hypnotic.

picogram (pg): unit of weight equivalent to 10^{-12} gram.

pituitary gland: tiny gland located at the base of the brain which controls hormone production in other endocrine glands.

placebo: "sugar pill" (a preparation with no medicinal properties) given as medicine for its anticipated effects.

premenstrual syndrome (PMS): variety of physical and emotional symptoms a woman may experience prior to menstruation.

progesterone: female sex hormone secreted by the corpus luteum, that prepares the uterus for pregnancy.

Prozac: trademark for the drug fluoxetine hydrochloride; used to treat depression.

sebaceous glands: glands of the skin which secrete a fatty substance to lubricate the skin.

surgical menopause: onset of menopause caused by the surgical removal of the ovaries.

Taxol: trade name for the drug paclitaxel; antitumor agent being used investigationally for the treatment of carcinomas and melanomas in the ovaries.

testis: male reproductive gland contained within the scrotum that produces sperm; typically found in pairs.

testosterone: male sex hormone produced in the testes, responsible for male secondary sex characteristics.

thrombophlebitis: formation of a blood clot in a blood vessel resulting in inflammation of the vein and partial or complete blocking of the blood vessel.

thymus: gland made up mostly of lymphoid tissue that aids in the development of the body's immune system.

thyroid: gland located in the neck that secretes hormones which play a major role in regulating the metabolic rate.

thyroxine: iodine-containing amino acid used to treat thyroid disorders.

Valium: trade name for the drug diazepam; tranquilizer used to treat tension and anxiety.

Bibliography

CHAPTER 1

Maddox, M.A. "Women at Midlife." *Nursing Clinics of North America* 1992;27(4):959–69.

Redmond, G. *The Good News About Women's Hormones.* Warner Books, 1995.

Sever, C.A. *It's Okay to Take Estrogen.* Eclectic Books, 1995.

CHAPTER 2

Burnett, R.G. *Menopause: All Your Questions Answered.* Contemporary Books, 1987.

Greendale, G.A., and Judd, H.L. "The Menopause: Health Implications and Clinical Management." *Journal of the American Geriatrics Society* 1993;41:426–36.

Landau, C., Cyr, M.G.H., and Moulton, A.W. *The Complete Book of Menopause: Every Woman's Guide to Good Health.* Grosset/Putnam, 1994.

Marsh, M.S., and Whitehead, M.I. "Management of Menopause." *British Medical Bulletin* 1992; 48(2):426–57.

Notelovitz, M., and Tonnessen, D. *Estrogen: Yes or No.* St. Martin's Paperbacks, 1993.

Speroff, L. "Menopause and Hormone Replacement Therapy." *Clinics in Geriatric Medicine* 1993;9(1):33–55.

CHAPTER 3

Barrett-Connor, E. "Estrogen and Estrogen-Progestogen Replacement: Therapy and Cardiovascular Diseases." *American Journal of Medicine* 1993;95(suppl 5A):40S–42S.

Binder, E.F., Birge, S.J., and Kohst, W.M., *et al.* "Effect of Endurance Exercise and Hormone Replacement Therapy on Serum Lipids in Older Women." *Journal of the American Geriatrics Society* 1996;44:231–36.

Grodstein, F., Stampfer, M.J., and Manson, J.E., *et al.* "Postmenopausal estrogen and progestin use and the risk of cardiovascular disease." *New England Journal of Medicine* 1996;335:453–61.

Manson, J.E. "Postmenopausal Hormone Therapy and Atherosclerotic Disease." *American Heart Journal* 1994;128:1337–43.

Schwartz, J., Freeman, R., and Frishman, W. "Clinical Pharmacology of Estrogens: Cardiovascular Actins and Cardioprotective Benefits of Replacement Therapy in Postmenopausal Women." *Journal of Clinical Pharmacology* 1995;35:314–29.

Watts, N.B., and Notelovitz, M. "Comparison of Oral Estrogens and Estrogens Plus Androgens on Bone Mineral Density, Menopausal Symptoms, and Lipid-lipoprotein Profiles in Surgical Menopause." *Obstetrics and Gynecology* 1995;85(4):529–37.

Wilkes, H.C., Vickers, M.R., and Browne, W., *et al.* "Randomized comparison of oestrogen versus oestrogen plus progestogen hormone replacement therapy in women with hysterectomy." *British Medical Journal* 1996; 312(1):473–78.

CHAPTER 4

Coope, J.K.M., and Coope, J.R. "HRT, A General Practice Approach: How to Reach the Most Vulnerable." *British Journal of Clinical Practice* 1996;50(1):40–43.

Dennison, E., and Cooper, C. "The Epidemiology of Osteoporosis." *British Journal of Clinical Practice* 1996;50(1):33–36.

Grey, A.B., Stapleton, J.P., and Evans, M.C., *et al.* "Effect of Hormone Replacement Therapy on Bone Mineral Density in Postmenopausal Women with Mild Primary Hyperparathyroidism." *Annals of Internal Medicine* 1996;125(5): 360–66.

Liberman, U.A., Weiss, S.R., and Broll, J., *et al.* "Effects of Oral Alendronate on Bone Mineral Density and the Incidence of Fractures in Postmenopausal Osteoporosis." *New England Journal of Medicine* 1995;33(22):1437–43.

Lindsay, R. "Hormone Replacement Therapy for Prevention and Treatment of Osteoporosis."

American Journal of Medicine 1993;95(suppl 5A): 5A37S–39S.

Miller, P.D. "Critical Drug Appraisal: Etidronate Intermittent Cyclic Therapy for Postmenopausal Osteoporosis." *British Journal of Clinical Practice* 1996;50(1):23–31.

Rowe, R. "Preventive Strategies: Is Current Clinical Practice Effective for Bones?" *British Journal of Clinical Practice* 1996;50(1):47–49.

Sambrook, P.N. "The Treatment of Postmenopausal Osteoporosis." *New England Journal of Medicine* 1995;33(22):1495–96.

Shanley, F. "Osteoporosis: Patient workup shows not all cases are postmenopausal." *Geriatrics* 1993;48(10):21.

CHAPTER 5

Berga, S.L. "Hormonal Management of the Sick Menopausal Woman." *Obstetrics and Gynecology Clinics of North America* 1994;21(2):231–44.

Evans, M.P., Fleming, K.C., and Evans, J.M. "Hormone Replacement Therapy: Management of Common Problems." *Mayo Clinic Proceedings* 1995;70:800–805.

Judd, H.L., Mebane-Sims, I., and Legault, C., *et al.* "Effects of Hormone Replacement Therapy on Endometrial History in Postmenopausal Women." *Journal of the American Medical Association* 1996;275(5):370–75.

Kritz-Silverstein, D., and Barrett-Connor, E. "Long-Term Postmenopausal Hormone Use,

Obesity, and Fat Distribution in Older Women." *Journal of the American Medical Association* 1996;275(1):46–49.

Lufkin, E.G., and Ory, S.J. "Relative Value of Transdermal and Oral Estrogen Therapy in Various Clinical Situations." *Mayo Clinic Proceedings* 1994;69:131–35.

Maddox, M.A. "Women at Midlife." *Nursing Clinics of North America* 1992;27(4):959–69.

Mort, E.A. "Clinical Decision-Making in the Face of Scientific Uncertainty: Hormone Replacement Therapy as an Example." *Journal of Family Practice* 1996;42(2):147–51.

Nachtigall, L.E. "Comparative Study: Replens Versus Local Estrogen in Menopausal Women." *Fertility and Sterility* 1994;61(1):178–80.

Reeve, J. "Future Prospects for Hormone Replacement Therapy." *British Medical Bulletin* 1992;48(2):438–68.

Stumpf, P.G., and Trolice, M.P. "Compliance Problems with Hormone Replacement Therapy." *Obstetrics and Gynecology Clinics of North America* 1994;21(2):219–29.

Thorneycroft, I.H. "Practical Aspects of Hormone Replacement Therapy." *Progress in Cardiovascular Diseases* 1995;38(3):243–55.

Udoff, L., Langenberg, P., and Adashi, E.Y. "Combined Continuous Hormone Replacement Therapy: A Critical Review." *Obstetrics and Gynecology* 1995;86(2):306–16.

CHAPTER 6

Adami, H., and Persson, I. "Hormone Replacement and Breast Cancer: A Remaining Controversy?" *Journal of the American Medical Association* 1995;274(1):178–79.

Barrett-Conner, E. "Risks and Benefits of Replacement Estrogen." *Annual Review of Medicine* 1992;43:239–51.

Colditz, G.A., Hankinson, S.E., and Hunter, D.J., *et al.* "The Use of Estrogens and Progestins and the Risk of Breast Cancer in Postmenopausal Women." *New England Journal of Medicine* 1995; 332:1589–93.

Daly, E., Vessey, M.P., and Hawkins, M.M., *et al.* "Risk of venous thromboembolism in users of hormone replacement therapy." *Lancet* 1996; 348:977–80.

Grodstein, F., Stampfer, M.J., and Manson, J.E., *et al.* "Postmenopausal Estrogen and Progestin Use and the Risk of Cardiovascular Disease." *New England Journal of Medicine* 1996;335:453–61.

Harding, C., Knox, W.I., and Faragher, E.B. "Hormone replacement therapy and tumour grade in breast cancer: prospective study in screening unit." *British Medical Journal* 1996; 312:1646–47.

Harris, R.E., Namboodiri, K.K., and Farrar, W.B., *et al.* "Hormone Replacement Therapy and Breast Cancer Risk." *Journal of the American Medical Association* 1996;275(15):1158.

Hazzard, W.R., Bierman, E.L., and Blass, J.P., *et*

al. Practices of Geriatric Medicine and Gerontology. McGraw-Hill, 1990.

Healy, B. *A New Prescription for Women's Health: Getting the Best Medical Care in a Man's World.* Viking, 1996.

Hulka, B.S., and Stark, A.T. "Breast Cancer: Cause and Prevention." *Lancet* 1995;346(8979): 883–87.

Jick, H., Berby, L.E., and Myers, M.W., *et al.* "Risk of hospital admission for idiopathic venous thromboembolism among users of postmenopausal oestrogens." *Lancet* 1996;348: 981–83.

Lark, S.M. *The Estrogen Decision Self-Help Book.* Celestial Arts, 1996.

McPherson, K. "Breast Cancer and Hormonal Supplements in Postmenopausal Women." *British Medical Journal* 1995;311(7007):699–700.

Neven, P., and DeMaylder, X. "Hormonal interventions and cancer risk." *Lancet* 1995; 346(suppl):S8.

Reichman, J. *I'm Too Young to Get Old: Health Care for Women After Forty.* Random House, 1996.

Smith, H.O., Kammerer-Doak, D.N., and Barbo, D.M., *et al.* "Hormone Replacement Therapy in the Menopause: A Pro Opinion." *Cancer Journal Clinics* 1996;46:343–63.

Stanford, J.L., Weiss, N.S., and Voigt, L.F., *et al.* "Combined Estrogen and Progestin Hormone Replacement Therapy in Relation to Risk of Breast Cancer in Middle-aged Women." *Journal of the American Medical Association* 1995;274: 137–42.

Stefanick, M.L., Legault, C., and Tracy, R.P., *et al.* "Distribution and Correlates of Plasma Fibrinogen in Middle-Aged Women." *Arteriosclerosis, Thrombosis, and Vascular Biology* 1995;15:2085–93.

Tang, M., Jacobs, D., and Stern, Y., *et al.* "Effect of oestrogen during menopause on risk and age at onset Alzheimer's disease." *Lancet* 1996; 348;429–32.

Wallis, L.A. "Hormone Replacement Therapy: Decision-Making in an Age of Uncertainty." *Journal of the American Medical Women's Association* 1992;47(6):225–29.

CHAPTER 7

Berman, R.S. "Compliance of women in taking estrogen replacement therapy." *Journal of Women's Health* 1996;5:213–20.

Coope, J.K.M., and Coope, J.R. "HRT, A General Practice Approach: How to Reach the Most Vulnerable." *British Journal of Clinical Practice* 1996;50(1):39–43.

Mort, E.A. "Clinical decision-making in the face of scientific uncertainty: hormone replacement therapy as an example." *Journal of Family Practice* 42(2):147–51.

Reeve, J. "Future prospects for hormone replacement therapy." *British Medical Bulletin* 1992; 48(2):458–68.

Stumpf, P.G., and Trolic, M.P. "Compliance Problems with Hormone Replacement Therapy." *Obstetrics and Gynecology Clinics of North America* 1994;21(2):219–29.

CHAPTER 8

Lichtman, R. "Perimenopausal and postmenopausal hormone replacement therapy." *Journal of Nurse Midwifery* 1996;41:195–210.

McGuffey, E.C. "Treating Hot Flashes." *American Pharmacist* 1995; NS35:14–17.

Rosenberg, L. "Hormone Replacement Therapy: The Need for Reconsideration." *American Journal of Public Health* 1993;83(12):1670–73.

CHAPTER 9

Healy, B. *A New Prescription for Women's Health: Getting the Best Medical Care in a Man's World.* Viking, 1996.

Jacobowitz, R.S. *One-Hundred and Fifty Most-Asked Questions About Menopause: What Women Really Want to Know.* William Morrow, 1996.

Kemper, D.W., McIntosh, K.E., and Roberts, T.M. *Healthwise Handbook.* Healthwise, 1991.

Lark, S.M. *The Estrogen Decision Self-Help Book.* Celestial Arts, 1996.

Murray, M.T. *Menopause: How You Can Benefit From Diet, Vitamins, Minerals, Herbs, Exercise, and Other Natural Methods.* Prima Publishing, 1994.

Reichman, J. *I'm Too Young to Get Old: Health Care For Women After Forty.* Random House, 1996.

Vickery, D.M., and Fries, J.F. *Take Care of Yourself.* Addison-Wesley, 1994.

Resources

There are numerous organizations and associations that provide information about menopause, HRT, and alternative treatments. All you have to do is contact them and ask for help. In this chapter, you will find an extensive listing of menopause referral and education resources—including government agencies, books, and a guide to locating medical information on the Internet.

ORGANIZATIONS THAT PROVIDE INFORMATION OR SUPPORT

American Academy of Family Physicians
8880 Ward Parkway
Kansas City, MO
64114-2797
Tel: 800-944-8000
Fax: 816-822-0580

American Association of Sex Educators, Counselors, and Therapists
Post Office Box 238
Mount Vernon, IA 52314
Tel: 319-895-8407

The American College of Obstetricians and Gynecologists (ACOG)
Office of Public Information
409 12th Street Southwest
Washington, DC 20024-2218
Tel: 202-484-3321
Fax: 202-479-6826

American Dietetic Association
216 West Jackson Boulevard
Suite 800
Chicago, IL 60601
Tel: 312-899-0040

American Fertility Society
1209 Montgomery Highway
Birmingham, AL 35216
Tel: 205-978-5000

American Medical Association (AMA)
515 North State Street
Chicago, IL 60610
Tel: 312-464-4818

American Medical Women's Association (AMWA)
801 North Fairfax Street
Suite 400
Alexandria, VA 22314
(703) 838-0500

Food and Drug Administration (FDA)
5600 Fisher's Lane
Rockville, MD 20857
Tel: 301-827-2410

HERS Foundation
Hysterectomy Educational Resources and Services
422 Bryn Mawr Avenue
Bala Cynwyd, PA 19004
Tel: 610-667-7757

Menopause News
2074 Union Street
San Francisco, CA 94123
Tel: 415-567-2368
Tel: 800-241-MENO

Midlife Women's Network
5129 Logan Avenue
Minneapolis, MN 55419
Tel: 800-886-4354
email: mdlfwoman@aol.com

National Council on Aging
600 Maryland Avenue Southwest
West Wing 100
Washington, DC 20024
Tel: 202-479-1200

National Health Information Center
Post Office Box 1133
Washington, DC 20013
Tel: 800-336-4797

The National Institute on Aging
Post Office Box 8057
Gaithersburg, MD 20898-8057
Tel: 800-222-2225

National Osteoporosis Foundation
2100 M Street Northwest
Washington, DC 20037
Tel: 202-223-2226

National Women's Health Hotline
Tel: 800-222-4767

The North American Menopause Society
University Hospitals
Department of Ob/Gyn
Post Office Box 94527
Cleveland, OH 44101-4527
Tel: 216-844-8748

The Older Women's League
666 11th Street Northwest
Suite 700
Washington, DC 20001
Tel: 202-783-6686

Seasons Magazine
100 Avenue of the Americas, 8th Floor
New York, NY 10013
Tel: 800-444-0494

Sexuality Information and Education Council of the United States
130 West 42nd Street
Suite 350
New York, NY 10036
Tel: 212-819-9770

ORGANIZATIONS THAT PROVIDE INFORMATION ON ALTERNATIVE THERAPIES

The American
  Association of
  Naturopathic
  Physicians
Post Office Box 20386
Seattle, WA 98102
Tel: 206-323-7610

The American Holistic
  Medical Association
4101 Lake Boone Trail,
  #201
Raleigh, NC 26707
Tel: 919-787-5146

American Menopause
  Foundation, Inc.
Madison Square Station
Post Office Box 2013
New York, NY 10010
Tel: 212-475-3107

The Herb Research
  Foundation
1007 Pearl Street
Suite 200
Boulder, CO 80302
Tel: 303-449-2265

National Center for
  Homeopathy
801 North Fairfax Street
Suite 306
Alexandria, VA 22314
Tel: 703-548-7790

National Institutes of
  Health
Office of Alternative
  Medicine
Building 31, Room 5B-38
9000 Rockville Pike
Bethesda, MD 20892
Mailstop 22182
Tel: 301-402-2466

National Institutes of
  Health
Office on Research on
  Women's Health
Building 1, Room 201
9000 Rockville Pike
Bethesda, MD 20892
Tel: 301-402-1770

National Institutes of Health
Women's Health Initiative
Federal Building, Room 6A09
9000 Rockville Pike
Bethesda, MD 20892
Tel: 800-549-6636

Transitions for Health
621 Alder Street Southwest
Suite 900
Portland, OR 97205
Tel: 800-888-6814

BOOKS ON MENOPAUSE, HRT, AND RELATED TOPICS

There are more books available today on menopause and its management—the physiology of menopause, the advantages and disadvantages of hormone replacement therapy, and other menopause management techniques—than ever before. Many of the following are available at the public library. Others can be ordered through booksellers.

Acupressure for Women, C. Bauer. The Crossing Press, 1987.

American Medical Association Pocket Guide to Calcium, the American Medical Association. Random House, 1995.

The Change: Women, Aging, and the Menopause, G. Greer. Alfred A. Knopf, 1991.

The Complete Book of Menopause, S. Perry and K. O'Hanlan, M.D. Addison-Wesley, 1992.

The Complete Book of Menopause, C.C. Landau, Ph.D., M.G. Cyr, M.D., and A.W. Moulton, M.D. Berkley Publishing Group, 1994.

The Complete Guide to Women's Health, B.D. Shephard, M.D., and C.A. Shephard, R.N. Penguin, 1987.

The Estrogen Decision Self-Help Book, S. Lark, M.D. Celestial Arts, 1996.

Estrogen Replacement Therapy User's Guide, R.D. Gambrell, M.D. Essential Medical Information Systems, 1996.

Estrogen, L. Nachtigall, M.D., and J.R. Heilman. HarperCollins, 1995.

Estrogen: Yes or No, M. Notolovitz, M.D., Ph.D., and D. Tonnessen. St. Martin's Paperbacks, 1993.

The Family Guide to Homeopathy, A. Lockie. Hamilton, 1990.

Gentle Yoga, L. Bell and E. Seyfer. Celestial Arts, 1995.

The Good News about Women's Hormones, G. Remond, M.D. Warner Books, 1995.

The Healing Herbs, M. Castleman. Bantam, 1995.

Hormones, Hot Flashes, and Mood Swings, C. Gillespie, M.D. Harper & Row, 1994.

Hysterectomy: Before and After, W.B. Cutler, Ph.D. Harper & Row, 1990.

I'm Too Young to Get Old: Health Care for Women After Forty, J. Reichman, M.D. Times Books, 1996.

It's Okay to Take Estrogen: In Fact, Estrogen May Be Your Best Friend For Life, C.A. Sevener. Eclectic Publishing, 1995.

Love, Sex and Aging, E.M. Brecher and the Editors of Consumer Reports Books. Consumers Union, 1984.

Managing Your Menopause, W.H. Utian, M.D., and R. Jacobowitz. Fireside Books, 1990.

Menopause: All Your Questions Answered, R.G. Burnett, M.D. Contemporary Books, 1987.

The Menopause and Hormonal Replacement Therapy, edited by R. Sitruk-Ware and W.H. Utian. Marcel Dekker, 1991.

Menopause: A Midlife Passage, J. C. Callahan. Indiana University Press, 1993.

Menopause and Midlife, R. Wells and M.C. Wells. Tyndale House Publishers, 1990.

Menopause and Midlife Health, M. Notolovitz, M.D., Ph.D., and D. Tonnessen. St. Martin's Press, 1993.

Menopause and the Years Ahead, M.K. Beard, M.D., and L.R. Curtis, M.D. Fisher Books, 1991.

Menopause Clinical Concepts, S. London, M.D., and H.T. Chihal, M.D. Essential Medical Information Systems, 1995.

The Menopause, Hormone Therapy, and Women's Health. Diane Publishing, 1992.

Menopause: How You Can Benefit from Diet, Vitamins, Minerals, Herbs, Exercise, and Other Natural Methods, M.T. Murray, M.D. Prima Publishing, 1994.

Menopause, Naturally: Preparing for the Second Half of Life, S. Greenwood. Volcano Press, 1996.

The New Our Bodies, Ourselves, The Boston Women's Health Book Collective. Simon and Schuster, 1996.

A New Prescription for Women's Health: Getting the Best Medical Care in a Man's World, B. Healy, M.D. Viking, 1996.

The New Joy of Sex: A Gourmet Guide to Lovemaking for the Nineties, A. Comfort, M.D. Pocket Books, 1992.

One-Hundred and Fifty Most-Asked Questions About Menopause, R. Jacobowitz. William Morrow, 1996.

The Pause, L. Barbach, Ph.D. Dutton Books, 1993.

Preventing and Reversing Osteoporosis: Every Woman's Essential Guide, A.R. Gaby, M.D. Prima Publishing, 1995.

The Scientific Validation of Herbal Medicine, D.B. Mowry. Keats Publishing, 1990.

The Silent Passage, G. Sheehy. Simon and Schuster, 1992.

Stay Cool Through Menopause, M. Frisch, M.D. The Body Press, 1993.

Without Estrogen, D. Ito. Random House, 1994. For a free copy call 800-669-0156 or write to: Marketing Department, Planned Parenthood Federation of America, Inc., 810 Seventh Avenue, New York, N.Y. 10019.

THE INTERNET

Most of the major medical organizations have websites or homepages—which generally post information and provide links to other areas of interest—and there are educational forums on nearly every health or medical topic. Anyone with access to the Internet can download information on various topics, including menopause, hormone replacement therapy, alternative therapies, and other management techniques.

Online sites can also provide a network of support and encouragement in the form of newsgroups and chat rooms. Newsgroups are areas in which people provide information and answer questions; some of these exchanges occur in "real time." In a chat room, you can participate in an ongoing group conversation on just about any subject.

"Search engines," such as Altavista, Excite, WebCrawler, and Yahoo, make it possible to do Internet searches on specific topics. Once in a search engine, you can use menopause- or HRT-related search words. Using the word "menopause" as a search word will generate hundreds of "hits." You will probably wish to narrow down your search by using a combination of key words—for example, "menopause and hormone replacement therapy."

Be cautious when using the Internet as a source for medical knowledge. While many legimate organizations post information on the Internet, there are no guarantees that all the facts and recommendations that you find there will be sound. You may also find yourself the victim of some cleverly disguised sales pitches. It is always best to discuss what you discover on the Internet with your doctor.

Index

235

Expertly detailed, pharmaceutical guides
can now be at your fingertips
from U.S. Pharmacopeia

THE USP GUIDE TO MEDICINES
78092-5/$6.99 US/$8.99 Can

- More than 2,000 entries for both prescription
  and non-prescription drugs
- Handsomely detailed color insert

THE USP GUIDE
TO HEART MEDICINES
78094-1/$6.99 US/$8.99 Can

- Side effects and proper dosages for over 400
  brand-name and generic drugs
- Breakdown of heart ailments such as angina,
  high cholesterol and high blood pressure

THE USP GUIDE TO
VITAMINS AND MINERALS
78093-3/$6.99 US/$8.99 Can

- Precautions for children, senior citizens and
  pregnant women
- Latest findings and benefits of dietary supplements

"REQUIRED READING FOR ANYONE FACING CANCER"
Harmon Eyre, M.D.,
Deputy Executive Vice President,
AMERICAN CANCER SOCIETY

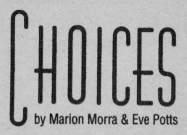

CHOICES
by Marion Morra & Eve Potts

COMPLETE • COMPREHENSIVE • RELIABLE
AUTHORITATIVE • REASSURING
DEFINITIVE • COMPASSIONATE • ESSENTIAL

Recommended by health care professionals nationwide, **CHOICES** is *the* leading sourcebook for cancer patients and their families—a unique and invaluable reference presenting important, up-to-date information in an accessible, easy-to-use format.

77620-0/ $15.00 US/ $20.00 Can

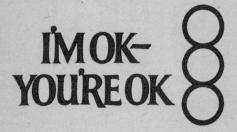